WILL OF IRON

WILL OF IRON

A Champion's Journey;
A Strategy for Fitness

Peter N. Nielsen

with Tom Ferguson

Momentum Books Ltd.
Ann Arbor

Cover photo by Rick Dinoian

Manufactured in the United States of America

1995   1994   1993   1992   5   4   3   2   1

Momentum Books, Ltd.
210 Collingwood, Suite 106
Ann Arbor, Michigan 48103
U.S.A.

ISBN 1-879094-19-3

Library of Congress Cataloging-in-Publication Data

Nielsen, Peter, 1961–
    Will of iron : a champion's journey—a strategy for fitness /
Peter Nielsen.
        p.   cm.
    ISBN 1-879094-19-3 (pbk.) : $14.95
    1. Exercise. 2. Physical fitness. 3. Health. I. Title.
RA781.N547   1992
613.7—dc20   92-27532
                                                         CIP

To Pete and Marie,
who gave me my good name;

and to Cindy,
who accepted it

Contents

Author's Preface

In life there is always opportunity. Sometimes we see it, sometimes we are too afraid to see it. Usually our fear is because opportunity means facing up to change.

At the time I didn't realize it, but as I look back now I see I was blessed with the opportunity to be a vehicle to touch the lives of many people. These are people of every sort—from persons with physical handicaps or serious challenges to meet, to top-rank athletes who have attained the pinnacle of performance in their fields.

It has always been my desire to help people learn from the experiences of others—and from the mistakes made by other people, including me. One lesson I learned painfully was that opportunity is adversity turned inside out. I discovered that when you are in a situation that can't be avoided but must be dealt with, it is the attitude we take that permits us, as William Faulkner said, not only to endure but to prevail.

Those challenges, those bad moments in life are our opportunities to make something more and better of ourselves. For me, my response to adversity took the form of building for myself a healthier life style. Much of what I discovered on that journey was learned from others.

But as much as I have wanted to share these insights and concepts with others, I realized long ago that I was unable to do it alone.

I wanted to light in others the same spark that had been kindled in me, the spark that saved my life. It was my great good fortune to meet up with Tom Ferguson, a person with the skill and determination to wade through the 31 years of my life and shape it into the story in these pages. His talent is considerable and is exceeded only by his qualities as a person. If this book speaks to you or touches you in any way—and I fervently hope that it does—then we both owe thanks to my collaborator, and my friend, Tom Ferguson.

P.N.N.
September 1992

Introduction

I don't look the same as someone who spends his life behind a desk or on a couch, smokes, eats 18 cheeseburgers a week and hasn't lifted anything heavier than a double martini in 15 years. More importantly, I don't *feel* the same. I get 24 good hours out of almost every day.

It's fascinating, and sad, that the average person probably considers me to be a freak.

That's because I pay serious attention to this one and only, fragile frame that I'll be living in from cradle to grave. Because I'm more aware of what I eat than I am of what's going to be on television tonight. Because I take better care of myself than of my dog—though Angel (she's a strong but gentle bull mastiff) lives a very good life. And because I'm a *bodybuilder*.

Well, I'm not a freak. And I'm not writing this book to convince you that every American should be down at the gym this afternoon doing double sets of curls with 50-pound dumbbells. You don't have to be a gym rat to be healthy and fit.

I'm writing this book because it pains me that in a society where "quality of life" and "quality time" have been buzz phrases for a decade or more, there is so little quality in most Americans' physical condition. It also pains me that human nature seems to require crisis before action—a fatal crash before a street light is installed, or a coronary before the junk food and the cigarettes get tossed aside. A near-fatal disease at a very young age gave me my own big-time wakeup call.

My main concern in writing this book has nothing to do with athleticism, or with muscular bodies than can be oiled up and displayed on a stage. It has everything to do with all the more important things that are affected by our physical condition. A short list, in no particular order, might include career, family life, sex life, longevity, self-esteem and earning power. In other words, every single thing that every self-help guru ever has proposed to improve for you.

Like any honest guru, my goal is to help you light your own inner fire—because of all the thousands of things that no one else can do for you, physical fitness is at the very top of the list. Fitness starts in your own mind, and is achieved in your own body. You can buy a personal trainer (and I honestly believe myself to be one of the best), but he cannot do the exercise for you. He cannot spoonfeed you your meals. He cannot be with you 24 hours a day to keep that motivational pilot light lit at the front of your brain. You have to make your own decision to *live,* instead of flushing your health down the toilet and dragging through life in an impaired body.

So let's get the Hans-and-Franz stuff out of the way from the get-go, and get on to more important things.

Ever play golf? The difference between Jack Nicklaus's backswing and yours is probably about the same as the difference between your pectorals and mine. I'm a pro. I've been fine-tuning my body for 15 years. I'm *supposed* to have unusual definition in my musculature. Jack Nicklaus is a pro. He's *supposed* to tap that little ball into the hole with unusual regularity.

Millions of people will sit for hours and watch the best golfers tap a little white ball. But there's something about a seriously developed body that, just by walking into a room, can trigger all kinds of bizarre reactions.

"He has a real narcissism problem."

"He's got more biceps than brains."

"He bought it at the drugstore."

Those deficiencies are sprinkled across the entire population, if you ask me. Even among people with small biceps.

A narcissist? I work just as hard at keeping my ego properly channeled as I do at lifting weights and monitoring my nutrition. Right now I'm putting more effort into—and getting more satisfaction from—helping other people get and stay fit than I ever put into my own training.

Barbells for brains? I'm not here to tell you that being fit will make you a genius. But the zest for life and the confidence that come with fine-tuning your body will most definitely help your career, no matter what you do. I successfully operate several businesses, fulfill a busy public-speaking schedule, do a fitness and health segment on TV news twice a week, and act as national spokesman in the campaign against a serious disease. I run out of clock, not out of gas.

As for drugs, I have a serious attitude on the subject. I got into this sport of bodybuilding to save my life, not to lose it. My gym is filled with trophies I won "clean" before retiring seven years ago. The main reason I came out of retirement in 1991 was that my sport finally has a sanctioning body that administers blood, urine and polygraph tests to all competitors. I always "walked what I talked"; now I can prove it.

My gym is filled with bodybuilders of both sexes and numerous ages, shapes and sizes. I think the range of clientele would stagger your mind. We have major-league hockey and basketball players, some media types, salesmen and saleswomen, blue-collar workers and professionals. Some pay the fee out of their walking-around money; some have to budget for the privilege of sweating.

Yes, some have musculature that requires them to seek custom tailors. But others would never stand out in a crowd—which is exactly their goal.

Tara Terrell, for instance, is a bodybuilder. She has lupus. Tara works out almost every day. She doesn't want to build a freak physique. She just wants to get her health back, to be mainstream.

Chuck Robertson is a successful businessman, the owner of a swimming pool company. He has a very rare, very debilitating disease that is attacking all of his muscles—even his tongue. He works out constantly to fight the atrophy, to keep the disease in remission. Chuck is a bodybuilder, one of the gutsiest I've ever met.

So if you take a look at the bodybuilding scene, the reality is that there are *two* stereotypes—one group of bodies that you more or less had pictured, and one group of bodies that you probably didn't.

Unfortunately, most bodybuilders fit one stereotype or the other: advanced practitioners of the sport, or fragile human beings who have found that their last, best chance lies in a serious physical regimen.

Either way, they are *building* their *bodies*. Getting healthier. Raising confidence and self-esteem.

Nothing freakish about that.

And if I get a little preachy, that's what I'm here to preach. Fitness. Plain and simple.

If you want to be a serious bodybuilder, that's great. You'll learn a lot in this book, including some bona fide secrets of a champion. But you can get a lot out of this book, too, *if you never do set foot in a gym.*

For one thing, gyms don't have a patent on exercise. Or even on bodybuilding. I worked out at home for a year and a half before setting foot in a gym. And competitive bodybuilding, contrary to what you might think, is just as much a matter of nutrition and mental toughness as it is a matter of pumping iron. I'm 31, working out less than two hours a day, and still competing at the highest levels in open professional company. Every check I take home now comes *more* from the kitchen than from the gym, *more* from the brain than from the sweat glands.

My gym, by the way, has a mile-long name. But the words were all important to me, so I put 'em all in: Peter Nielsen's Eye of the Tiger Total Fitness Center. My own name I had to use, of course. *Eye of the Tiger* means something very special to me, and potentially to you, as you'll see in a later chapter.

Total Fitness Center is not a unique phrase, but we absolutely mean every letter of it. Some of our customers just want to come in and lift weights. That's OK. But I also offer nutrition counseling, advice on training programs and sometimes just a good talk on the self-discipline it takes to bring out your best. Next-door we have an aerobics center; and, yes, I try to get even our best lifters involved over there. Why? Because if you can bench-press the Empire State

Building but you're sucking air walking up two flights of steps, then you haven't accomplished much, have you?

So it's a *total* package, this business of fitness, just like life is a total package. If you get obsessed with pumping iron, you *are* a musclehead. My wife, my family, my religion, my health, my friends, my fitness message, my businesses, my athletic competition—that's my priority list right now. I've never been happier.

Everybody puts his or her life in a package. Things can get crowded in there, right? Whatever it is that you do for a living seems to take up so much space. A friend of mine is into computers. He showed me a software program that will take a data file and compress it so your disk will hold umpteen more files and work more efficiently besides. And that, my friend, is what fitness will do for *your* total package. The irony is that most of us don't include a fitness program because we think there is no room.

That's why most Americans fall somewhere into the vast, flabby middle ground between those two bodybuilding stereotypes. Fitness is something they want to be involved in, but can't seem to make time for. They make well-intentioned but humorous little stabs at it—ordering a meatloaf sandwich on whole wheat instead of white, or eating frozen yogurt instead of ice cream in front of the TV. They're *thinking* about fitness, all right, but not very hard. *Some day* they'll do something about it.

"Some day" usually arrives after that first coronary, or when—middle-aged, 50 pounds overweight and barely functioning outside the brain—they discover that the image reflected in their spouse's eye is not exactly what it used to be.

The lucky ones respond sooner. They keep hearing about quality time, but when they find time they don't find much quality. They're too tired to play with the kids, or they come home from work too tired to go out to a movie. And, bless 'em, they decide to do something about it.

The fact is, if the average American treated his body half as well as he treats his car, he'd be a lot happier and healthier.

Think about it.

That hunk of metal in the driveway gets filled up with whatever grade of gasoline it needs to run at its best, no more and no less.

The first hint of a little sluggishness in the engine's performance and we rush it in for a tune-up. In fact, we maintain all moving parts regularly—even if no warning signs are present.

Appearance? Clean, well-defined lines that pop out and scream, "I'm at my best"? Well, we wash and polish that sheet metal as if our cars—and not our bright or bleary eyes—were the windows of our souls. More likely, we have somebody else do the washing and polishing.

Meanwhile, most Americans treat their own bodies like junkers, rustmobiles that they're just trying to get a few more miles out of. And in many cases, that's all they'll get.

At best, a junker will cough and wheeze up hills all day, then stagger home at night and plop in the garage. Wanna go for a spin? Not tonight. All out of gas.

That's an awful lot of car talk. But the analogy seems right, for a couple of reasons.

For one thing, I'm a Brooklyn boy transplanted to the Motor City. You can't live within 50 miles of Detroit without having cars on the brain.

For another thing, I've had my own intense love affairs with wheels—from the used Maverick that was my first and somehow best, to the Porsche 928 that I mistakenly thought was something a Mr. International Universe *had* to be driving. So I understand how 2,000 pounds of machinery dressed in red represents something more than a way to get from Point A to Point B. I even understand how those overpowered phallic symbols of my childhood came to be called *muscle* cars.

But all the ego riding on raised-letter $300 tires is just one example of where we have our priorities and our goals seriously mixed up.

God gives us just one model year—the one that we're born in. There are no trade-ins. And, with apologies to the transplant surgeons, spare parts won't make up for bad maintenance.

It's a national tragedy that there are far more junkers on our couches than in our garages.

It's great to have all those trophies cluttering up my gym, it's great to go on national TV, it's great to have companies give me endorsement money just because I've put in the sweat equity and discipline to fine-tune my body to its maximum. But I've got to tell you, these days you can go just halfway—a quarter of the way—down my road and still stand out in a crowd.

Maybe it's a wonder that we're as fit as we are. It used to be much easier, back before elevators and Nintendo and Big Macs. I guarantee you that if I could hop in a time machine and land in a crowd of 19th-Century farm workers, my arms wouldn't particularly look like anything special.

The bad news is that our kids are in even more desperate straits. And since the vigor of youth *temporarily* overcomes all kinds of fitness sins, we're talking about a real time bomb.

Our young people have been nuked all their lives with commercials for eating material. I hesitate to call it food. This stuff is to food what a billboard is to literature.

Almost straight from the cradle our kids sit in front of the TV and absorb hours of hype for breakfast stuff, most of which is the junkiest of junk foods. High-priced junk, at that.

Water? If the commercial media represented reality, the textbooks would say that the human body needs 15 glasses of beer and pop a day for survival.

Why am I not surprised that the teenager's *lunch* of choice contains more grams of fat than I eat in three or four days?

Put all that garbage in the stomach of a generation that gets its exercise playing video games and you have a blueprint for disaster. You think health-care costs are eating up an obscene part of our national treasure now? Wait a while.

The good news is that you can do something about all this gloom and doom. You can take care of your own body. You can't take care of your neighbor's. But you probably don't wash his car, either.

As for your kids, well, better people than me have failed while trying to get their children to do the right thing. But getting your own package together won't hurt. Be honest. What do your kids see *you* eating? How much exercise do they see *you* getting? You *are* a role model, even if it doesn't often seem that way.

Bodybuilding? Maybe. I recommend it for almost anybody. And we'll talk about it a lot in this book. I *am* a serious bodybuilder. I love the sport. In fact, I owe my life to bodybuilding, as you will see. But you don't have to play football to read about that sport, and I think you'll do yourself a lot more good reading these pages.

Part One is my story, some of which is painful and not very pretty. I fit that second, lesser-known stereotype. I'm not sure any bodybuilding champion ever emerged from a frame as fragile, malfunctioning and physically and emotionally scarred as the body I lived in in 1976. And my entrepreneurial career didn't start out much better.

Talking about my own adversities in this book is *not* an ego trip. When life turns out to be very good for someone who thought he was dealt the crummiest of hands, then he *owes* the telling of the tale. We all have adversities, and the things I learned about making negatives into positives can work for you, too.

Part Two will explain why I really mean it when I say the kitchen is my most important training room. You may never get into bodybuilding—or you may already be seriously into the sport. Either way, you'll want to know why *a single can* of diet pop six days before a competition will lose it for me. You'll want to know what different foods will and won't do for you, why timing your meals is important—and scores of other tips that are important to anyone who cares about his or her body.

Part Three is about sweat. There is no substitute for it—whether you're pumping iron, or walking, or exercising in your living room. The consumerist society keeps telling us to *get* things, but fitness is something you must *do*. I'll show you many different ways to do it, from designing a fitness program without spending a penny to a workout for a hard-core bodybuilder.

Part Four shows you how the mind, in the end, is your most powerful tool. Bodybuilding may be a muscle game, but it's the mind that wins the medals. That steely determination that gets every ounce of achievement possible from your body—the "intangible" that sportscasters talk about—really comes from the mind, of course, not the heart. And you *can* develop it. I'll show you how.

All four sections add up to a cookbook with one recipe, a recipe for *life*. You're the cook. How you use the recipe is up to you.

If you've ever spent any time in the kitchen, if you can cook anything that doesn't come in a box or a can, then you know a couple of things about recipes.

First, a good cook and a good recipe can combine for an infinite number of variations to fit differing resources, needs and tastes.

Second, you can't substitute whipping cream for cauliflower.

So open your mind, respect the integrity of the recipe, and find what works for you.

Part One

Scars and Barbells

1

Focus, Focus, Focus

Sometimes you get so focused you can't see straight.

I got that way in a fierce rain along the New Jersey Turnpike in November 1991.

Why was I so narrowly focused that for a minute I couldn't remember what life is about? So intent that my prized mental toughness almost got in the way of reality?

You have to understand: Physical fitness is my life, but body-building is my *sport*. For nearly seven years I had stayed away from it. And now, in 24 hours, I was going to be on the stage of the Park Theatre in New York, competing with top professionals from around the world.

On the plane from Detroit I was almost in a meditative mode. I'd image the theater stage and what I'd do there, and then I'd re-image it, over and over again. Sitting next to me must have been like sitting next to a log. One with lots of moss.

It's hard to say that what goes on in the last few days before a championship isn't self-absorption. It is. But it's not a deranged ego at work. Nobody would walk up to a linebacker putting on his game face just before the Super Bowl and say: "Excuse me, sir, but you seem to be a little self-absorbed." Putting on your game face for a professional bodybuilding competition is just as intense.

There are no teammates to bang helmets with, nobody to high-five. It's a lonely game where you train with your muscles and win with your mind. Your self is your whole team.

You want to pick out the winner at a bodybuilding competition? Forget the muscles. Up on that stage they've *all* got muscles. Look in the *eyes*. That's the window where you see whether the white-hot fire and the cool confidence have peaked together into a winning package. Focus. Focus. Focus.

I was realistic about my chances in this World Cup. Six and a half months isn't much training for a championship—especially when you've been away so long. But I was looking good. I felt good. If I stayed focused, I'd do OK.

The last time I had competed in New York I was a hometowner, a 23-year-old certified Adonis, the reigning Mr. International Universe, cruising the Big Apple glitz circuit. I posed in celebrity discos, dated beautiful women, schmoozed with the famous and near-famous and soon-to-be-famous on Julio Iglesias's yacht. In a steroid-tainted sport, I competed "clean"—and won it all. But away from the gym and off the bodybuilding stage I had become Mr. International Party Animal—so *unfocused* I couldn't see straight. It was time to escape from New York.

Michigan was where I put it back together, away from the glitz— and away from the sport I loved in its untainted form. By 1991 I had businesses and I had a TV job and I had all the speaking engagements I could handle. Fitness is teachable to any willing student, and I seek them out anywhere I can find them: in my gym, in schools, on TV, on videos, in the press. One restaurant in my suburban Detroit neighborhood even put a "Peter Nielsen recommends" section on its menu for people who want to think about what they eat.

Fitness is a *calling* to me. I talk it and I walk it. I keep myself healthy and incredibly in love with being alive. I help other people move in the same direction, and I'm constantly trying to find ways of reaching more people—especially kids—with the message. That's all I do. And in a little glimpse of heaven, I make a good living at the same time.

So why come out of retirement at age 30? Why this trip to New York?

For one thing, I do love the sport. The competition. The confidence to walk up there alone and say: "Here I am. I put in the sweat equity, the nutritional discipline, the mental toughness. I've taken the machine God gave me and tuned it to its absolute maximum. Do I win, or not?" I guess it's a special kick to win when God didn't seem to give you that much of a body to begin with.

For another thing, when you have a message for the public, it doesn't hurt to get a little international publicity, a few more pieces of metal to hang on the wall, one more credential.

For another thing, you can cash a check. This *is* professional competition. And the endorsement money and appearance money that goes with winning the big events dwarf the prize money itself.

But most important of all, a new group—the World Natural Bodybuilding Federation—finally had taken steps to get the monkey off bodybuilding's back. If you enter a WNBF event, you are certifiably clean. Your blood, your urine and your lie-detector test say so. No walking drugstores allowed in the winner's circle.

When I competed as a kid, I competed against steroids. *Most* of my competitors were on steroids. Some of them were my friends. Some still are.

But steroids angered me, disgusted me, made me feel dirty even if I didn't touch them. I won without the "juice," but the sleazeball image that steroids gave my sport was a heartbreaker. I absolutely couldn't believe what these guys were doing to their health in a game that supposedly was all about health.

Steroids kill. Even as a teenager, and even before the public awareness of the last decade, I knew what steroids will do to a body. I knew that while steroids built up muscle they tore down the liver, shrank testicles, did more bad things to a body than a mad scientist could imagine. And I had too much personal experience with a frail, diseased body to go down that path.

Nonetheless, a lot of people assumed that I found my muscles in a capsule or in a syringe. After all, I was a bodybuilder.

When I came out of retirement in 1991, I slipped down to Spartanburg, South Carolina, and won first place in the regional Mr. U.S.A. competition. I needed that trophy to qualify for the World Cup competition. A couple of *my own clients*—nice people who have seen me train, who know my life-style, who know what I think about drugs of *any* kind—were heard to say: "Hey, Peter must have had a little help, don't you think? I mean, winning Mr. U.S.A. that quick?"

That's how big my sport's monkey had become. And that's why the WNBF was an idea whose time was way past due. And that's why I was on a plane for New York.

My wife, Cindy, is a beautiful and talented graphics artist. When she married me earlier in 1991 she suddenly found that she was no longer an ad agency employee, but manager of a gym. Suddenly she was a chocaholic living with a guy whose idea of a good meal is oats, or egg whites, or broiled chicken breasts. She didn't fight it; she joined it. No problem.

Bodybuilding competition, though, was something new for Cindy. Mr. U.S.A., the first time she had seen me prep for an event, went smooth enough—even with the heightened training regimen and the six carefully planned meals a day. But New York and the World Cup started out as quite a different story. I was tense on the plane. And after we got off in Newark, she may have been having second thoughts about the whole deal. One minor screwup after another got in the way of all my focussing and made me even more of a bear. Unreasonable, grouchy, worthy of the classic slap upside the head.

Somebody gave us wrong directions on transport to the hotel. (Focus, Peter, focus.) A rent-a-car was supposed to be waiting. No rent-a-car. (Focus, Peter, focus.) It was pouring rain, and we had to find a bus to get to the car. (Focus, Peter, focus.)

By the time we made our way onto the freeway, peering through the windshield wipers, the delicate porcelain shell that I had put together was starting to show some hairline cracks. One nervous default from my dietary regimen, just one surrender to a handy can of diet pop, would be enough sodium to soften the hard-earned "cuts"—or definition—of my musculature and put my title hopes in the tank. Sloshing down the highway toward the city, I realized I was damned near in tears. Cindy had never seen me like this. In a few hours I would be taking a polygraph test, and I was not exactly a paragon of calm determination. What does that do to a polygraph test? I don't know. The tough mental focus was getting a little blurry.

Up ahead, though, flashing red lights cut through the rain. Traffic slowed to a crawl, and we eased past a couple of people who were not the least worried about staying focused. They weren't worrying about anything.

Right where the Turnpike splits to the Garden State Parkway, a car was wrapped around the ramp. An EMS crew was draping sheets over two human beings. Both were lying right on the road in pouring rain. It was obvious they were not alive.

We went past without saying a word.

A couple of miles later, a car was cruising down the shoulder, going 35 or 40 m.p.h. on three tires and a rim, sparks spitting from the rim into the slop, the driver hanging out the window because his wipers weren't working. This New Jersey madman was *focused* on getting to an exit.

I turned to Cindy and said, "It's just a bit *relative,* how I feel, isn't it?"

The cliche is "putting it in perspective." Cliche or not, I want to tell you that two miles of freeway put *everything* into perspective for me.

The accident shook me up. I almost got sick over seeing so much tragedy up close. But, for me, it was a negative/positive thing. Here I was getting all built up over nothing, over bad weather and rent-a-car foul-ups getting in the way of my mental preparation for a body-building competition. I was behaving about as smart as the guy flying along with three wheels and no wipers.

So I absolutely mellowed out. Focused, yes. Crazy, no.

For a few rainy minutes I had forgotten that, ultimately, adversity always has been my best friend.

And, as I always do when I screw up and feel sorry for myself, I remembered when I *really* felt sorry for myself—and what an incredible waste of time that was.

2

A World Turned Inside Out

Picture Bensonhurst in the '70s.

Say what? Yuh dunno Bensonhurst?

Sorry. Even today I sometimes forget that Brooklyn was never the center of the universe. It seemed to be back when I was growing up.

I lived in my grandmother's ancient six-unit apartment building from the time my parents brought me home, brand-new, until I got my own place when I was 19.

The streets of Brooklyn were the whole world to me. It's not like I'm old enough that I missed the TV revolution. But we spent a lot more time on the streets than we did watching the tube. So I didn't get any homogenized idea about what daily life was supposed to look like.

To me the heartbeat of America was Sixty-Seventh Street between Tenth and Eleventh avenues, right outside the building my mother's mother spent half a century paying for and where Frankie Puccio lived right across the hall. Out my door, knock on Frankie's door, and we already had a forward and a goalie (me) for a street hockey game. And we played *serious* street hockey.

I don't know what your image of Brooklyn street hockey is. But if it's anything like what my friends in the Midwest these days have in mind, you're way off base. We're not talking the Bowery Boys and a tin can and an old stick. We all had paper routes or we shined shoes, or both, and we went out and bought genuine equipment: pads, sticks—the whole nine yards, even the nets.

Sixty-Seventh Street is one-way. We'd put the hockey nets on rollers. Then we'd go at it and let traffic back up for a few minutes until somebody honked and yelled loud enough. Then we'd roll the nets aside, let the cars go by, and start checking and passing and shooting again.

We all went out and got plastic-tipped sticks, held them over the stove to bend them, then taught ourselves how to lift the puck. It was a street puck, solid plastic that took a lot of beating—and would give *you* a pretty good beating if you got hit with it.

I was always the goalie, but I taught myself how to use a curved stick anyway. One day, Anthony Fiotto was coming by on his way home from Catholic school, and those of us from McKinley Junior High were already out on the street playing. Anthony was standing talking to a girl he was trying to impress, and I decided to impress both of them.

"Hey Tony," I yelled. "Look at this. I can lift the puck!"

So Anthony looked at me, and I laid into a slap shot. It must have been a good one, because Anthony never moved. He took it on the chin and on the lip. Opened his face right up. He was standing there in his school uniform, with blood all over his face and his shirt and his tie, a total disaster. And the girl he was impressing just stood there with her jaw open.

We were all of us getting hurt, in one game or another. We were a real athletic bunch. Not on school teams, but in the neighborhood. We had Pony League baseball, but most of the action was right there on Sixty-Seventh Street. Street hockey, punchball, two-hand touch football—with the sidelines running from sewer to sewer.

Our touch football games were probably rougher than if we had suited up and played on a real field. I broke my nose playing touch. We'd mark the yard lines on Sixty-Seventh with chalk, then we'd go over the lines with a candle so they wouldn't disappear in the rain.

I was the only kid on the block without an Italian name. My father was Danish. That was all right, because my mother is as Italian as they come. I had a real fine Roman nose until it disappeared in that touch game, and a few other times.

The private clubs dotting the neighborhood were, as they say, well-connected. That's where I would shine shoes, starting around age nine or 10. Some of these guys would be loan sharks, some of them degenerate gamblers. I suppose I shined shoes for a hit man or two. Sometimes I'd come home with $11 or $12 in my pocket.

One time someone stole the jewels off the icons at Regina Pacis Church on Sixty-Fifth Street. Neighborhood talk put their value at $2 million. That's probably a little inflated, but they were worth more than money to the parish. The Gallo family and the Gambino family put out the word: Bring the jewels back within 24 hours, or else. No one ever said who took them, or what happened to the thieves, but in 24 hours the jewels were back on the statues.

This was a tough, tight-knit ethnic neighborhood. I got involved in a lot of fights. It wasn't because I had a chip on my shoulder. I certainly wasn't a bully. I was slim and short. Most of my girlfriends weighed a few pounds more than I did. The occasional fight just seemed to go with the turf. Like a lot of things, including the illness that almost killed me, I thought it was a part of growing up.

When I was 14, I got stabbed in the shoulder. It was just another fight, with a kid who was a troublemaker from the time he was in kindergarten. I don't know if I would have won the fight, but he made sure I didn't by stabbing me. I wanted to retaliate, but my Dad said: "Listen, somebody more stupid than you will take care of him someday. I call you stupid for lowering yourself to his level." It took eight years, but my Dad proved to be right. My sister called one day and said the neighborhood bully who had stabbed me was now a 22-year-old corpse, shot to death in a Brooklyn hallway.

There was a lot of well-publicized racial tension in Bensonhurst. If a black family moved into the neighborhood, a brick would go through their window—or a firebomb. Police cars got set on fire. Brotherhood among all human beings is something that has become important to me. But the things that disgust me now when I see them on TV, or in retrospect in my mind's eye, seemed in my youth to be just another part of the way things were.

Even in that climate, there was one kid at Fort Hamilton High who was to all of us neither black nor white, but simply *awesome*. Basketball was never my sport, partly because of my size, but I remember scrimmaging with this kid. Many people and places have been intimidating in my life. But trying to shoot hoops against Bernard King, even in a meaningless pick-up game, would rank near the top. It was fascinating to see someone who was *so good* at something. We all couldn't wait to see him get beyond high school, because it was just so obvious that he was going to the top.

I loved grade school and junior high. I got average grades or better, came home each afternoon to load up on Twinkies and milk and jelly junk, then went out onto Sixty-Seventh Street for the day's urban athletics. It was the only groove I knew, and it seemed just fine.

High school was another story.

When I got to Fort Hamilton High, in the 10th grade, I was right on track to make it through and meld into the neighborhood as an adult. I became a Bomber Jacket—we wore short leather flier's coats and wore our hair shorter than the other group, the Hippies. We caused minor problems, but we went to class. On the surface, except for being shorter and lighter than I should have been, I was pretty much your typical Bensonhurst adolescent. But this is exactly where my world started to tear apart.

For one thing, high school was even tougher than the streets of the neighborhood. It was not a pleasant place to be. For another thing, if you wanted to find some trouble—kids smoking marijuana, kids wanting to start a fight—the place to go was the boys' room at Fort Hamilton High. And sometime in the 10th grade, I began to need ever more frequent trips to the toilet.

There is no way to tell the story of my disease without talking about trips to the toilet, and about bodily functions. Maybe that's why so few people know about the disease, even though it is a potentially deadly affliction suffered by some 200,000 Americans. Ten times that suffer from other diseases of the lower digestive tract. It simply is not a popular or pleasant topic.

So consider this fair warning if you're reading while curled up with a bag of chips and a cola. You shouldn't be eating them anyway.

My parents thought I was just thin and on the scrawny side.

My friends thought I was just thin and on the scrawny side. Long after I should have known better—yearning in a teenaged panic to be normal—*I* thought I was just thin and on the scrawny side. My intestines began to tell me otherwise. At some point I went into denial because I was embarrassed to say I had the runs so often.

My mother, my father, my sister and I were crammed into a two-bedroom apartment with a single bathroom. Sometimes I would be in there for an hour, in distress, while an anxious line formed outside.

I lost so many half days at school that my teachers began to think I was avoiding class. At home, it got to be a case of: "Oh oh. It's Monday morning and Peter's going to have another excuse." The reality was I was sick. And even if I was willing to risk excusing myself from class so I could hustle down the hall, there was a real gauntlet to be run in any trip to the boys' room. Often I chose to stay home instead.

It's hard to explain, but just like many other aspects of growing up in Bensonhurst, I told myself: "Well, that's the way it is. That's the way it's going to be. That's me."

I still played street hockey or punchball every day—though I'd have to excuse myself too often. And afterward, when I should have been doing homework, I would sleep. Little cuts appeared in the skin around my eyes. The scrawny but athletic kid was experiencing serious fatigue. My mother was always having to wake me up for dinner.

My condition put stress on the family, which already was borderline dysfunctional. There was a lot of love in that apartment, but things weren't right.

My dad smoked—little Between the Acts cigars that he inhaled and left him waking up with a cough. And, after putting in a hard day at work, he drank too much. Not falling-down drunk, not to the point of abusing us; but too much to go through life without taking a serious toll on his body. He was a telephone lineman who would take me on wonderful hunting trips, a solid guy whose idea of a good time was to stop at a Flatbush bar at night and bend elbows with his friends. When I was 14, he enrolled me in karate school. I wasn't too thrilled, but it was perfect for Dad because karate school was right down the street from the Avenue U Bar. A year later, he had a 15-year-old son who was a runt, and who had taken to spending an hour at a time in the bathroom.

My sister was struggling with her own urban teenaged problems, trying to be a young woman while sharing her room with her brother.

My mother was protective of everyone, which circled back on her and sooner or later made her everybody's target. There was tension and there were shouting matches.

I internalized it all. Arguments were a good excuse to go take a nap.

Denial and reality met head-on one night that will stand forever, I hope, as the most embarrassing and frightening moment of my life.

I had saved up $900 from my paper route and from shining shoes. My Dad and Mom threw in another $500, which was enough to buy a Ford Maverick, my first and favorite car. A New York learner's permit allowed me to drive despite my age. It was more likely the Maverick than my Roman nose that got me a date with a girl I had been eyeing for weeks. With my wheels, a great night at the movies, and a visit to the diner, I was determined to make a first-class impression.

Something from the concession stand—popcorn, maybe, or candy—whipped my stomach like you would never believe. Driving away from the theater, with my date starting to get cozy and romantic, I was in agony and terror. I didn't know if I was going to be able to keep my insides under control. I told her I had a flat, pulled the Maverick over to the curb, and got out.

Away from the lights, dizzy, I started hemorrhaging. I could see the red flowing down the crease of my cream-colored pants, along with the contents of my bowels.

This, finally, was something that couldn't be denied. I was a 15-year-old kid who had just turned inside out, literally and figuratively, standing alongside a curb in Bensonhurst. I was street-smart, athletic, young and immortal. But the most vile contents of my body were drooling out onto the street.

I was in shock. *Literal* shock, and it seemed somehow logical that the thing to do was to get back inside my car. I did. My date grossed out and caught a cab. I drove home, snuck into the apartment and cleaned myself up. Then I went to my mother and said: "Mom, I've got a problem."

She took me to what seemed like two dozen doctors. I was tested for diseases I thought were extinct, or foreign, or only existed in bad movies. Malaria, leukemia, typhoid. I remember my mother getting upset because halfway through all the futile testing several of her friends insisted that I probably had tuberculosis. Medicine was well into the modern era in 1976, but it could not figure out what was wrong with me.

One day the phone rang and a doctor told my Mom to take my temperature, "right now while you're on the phone." The thermometer registered 99 degrees, and the doctor had his "Aha!" The lab had reported mononucleosis, the temperature confirmed it, and everybody was supposed to feel relieved.

My white cell count was abnormal, that was true. I did have mono. But I wasn't getting nutrients, and mono wasn't the real problem. We didn't know that, and we followed the standard drill.

I stayed home for three weeks, took a little medication, got my immune system functioning again, went back to school.

Boom! The same old bathroom symptoms returned, along with the chills.

We went through all the tests again, including upper and lower GI's, this time with an internist on Seventy-Fifth Street in Bay Ridge, a Dr. Imperato. Before I was through with him, this very wise man, since deceased, would tell me some important things in one of the most on-target, human, forceful speeches you will ever hear from the mouth of a medical doctor.

In mid-November, Dr. Imperato put me in Long Island University Hospital—which is in Brooklyn—for still more tests. I was supposed to be there for the weekend, and I was upset about it.

How can you explain that? Maybe a teenaged sense of immortality plus a little street macho add up to a sick kid who, even after baffling the medical establishment for a month and a half, resents being sent to the hospital. I went in with a chip on my shoulder.

When I came out nearly two months later, my whole body was about the size of a chip. And I wouldn't have to worry about going back to Fort Hamilton High again.

3

The Bridge

The doctors kept pulling at straws, and all the straws were somewhere on my body. The nurses started running out of places to draw blood. The lab started running out of new tests to try. The weekend in the hospital started to look more like permanent residency.

I was raised Catholic, and Christmas was my big holiday—gifts and snow and lights. After I'd been in the hospital almost a month, I kept asking if I'd be home for Christmas. And every day the docs would come through and say, "Looks good," or, "I don't know." And they kept taking tests.

Finally they decided that exploratory surgery would be necessary. Christmas was only a couple of days away, and I wasn't scheduled until after the holiday. Out the window I could see the snow and the lights of Brooklyn. I was genuinely messed up, in my head and somewhere in my abdomen.

The one diagnosis anybody was sure of was that I had an attitude problem, that the kid was maybe a dime short of a quarter. And Christmas is when I lost it.

It's a weird time to be in a hospital under any circumstances. Staff members have that holiday mood, and they have their little office parties like anyone else. You see Christmas trees in the wards and decorations hanging maybe 20 feet from where somebody has a few hours left to live. And when the holiday itself comes, a lot of the regulars get some well-deserved time off.

I grew almost accustomed to being a sort of living lab sample, but only for my regular cast of examiners. On or about Christmas 1976 I was put on display for a whole new group of pokers and prodders and viewers. The interns—most of whom spoke only broken English—were in command.

The curtain closed around my bed and the chief intern was presenting me and my puzzling condition to six of his colleagues. They put flashlights on me, and they asked each other questions as if I were dead—or at least under anesthesia. They wanted to do some kind of exam, wanted me to drop my hospital gown for a whole new set of strangers. One of them reached to touch me and I let loose.

"Out! Out!" I yelled. "The interview is *over*! Get the hell out!"

I don't know who was exhibiting the scummier behavior, me or them. I think it was them. Take your poodle to the vet and the patient will get more respect.

I shut down emotionally and physically. The staff let the sleeping dog lie and didn't bother to come and take blood that night.

Dr. Imperato, the internist who had sent me to the hospital and ultimately to the surgeons, came to my room. The kid from Brooklyn was still struggling to hold a chip on his shoulder, still trying to be cocky and macho, still internalizing so much emotion. I was a pouting child with clenched fists and crossed arms.

He sat on my bed and turned my head away from the cartoons or whatever I was watching on TV.

"I want you to understand," he said. "You're a very sick kid. Two things can happen. You can either feel sorry for yourself, or you can start showing some emotions and be a human being. You can stop the denial and you can grow up."

At that moment I hated this doctor who had put me in the hospital for a weekend that refused to end. He went on.

"You know what your problem is? You hold everything in. It's OK. You can cry." I don't know if "tough love" theory was being talked up back then, but Dr. Imperato knew what he was doing. He went on antagonizing me.

Finally I just let out the biggest cry—because I was scared to death. I was entrapped within my body, which had something seriously wrong with it, and nobody knew what it was.

The exploratory surgery solved that problem. It turned out to be more than exploratory, in fact. I left the operating room with a foot and a half of my large intestine missing. I had something called Crohn's disease—had it from the day I was born and will have it until the day I die.

In a way it was a relief, finally, to have a name on which to hang all this misery. But after so much time even the solution to the puzzle seemed unreal. So many questions. Hundreds of thousands of people have this unheard-of disease? I have it bad enough to fade away to less than 100 pounds approaching my 16th birthday? Nobody can find it for three months, and on the day it's found they spread my guts on an operating table and don't put all of them back in?

Yes. Yes. Yes.

I also was discovered—belatedly—to have a lactose intolerance. Want to start spending your days in the bathroom again, young man? Try having some milk or some cheese. Forget having ice cream. And, for sure, don't be thinking that you can eat pizza.

Double whammy. But the lactose intolerance, devastating as it was to a teenager who thought junk food and pizza were the staff of life, was nothing more than an inconvenience. And, besides, you could probably cheat occasionally, right? This Crohn's, however, was something else.

Besides losing a chunk of intestine, I came out of surgery with stitches in my rectum to close fissures that had ripped open from so much distress. I woke up wearing an ostomy bag to capture body waste. Maybe we'll be able to take it off when the torn tissue heals, the doctors said. Or maybe not.

Crohn's is a mystery in nearly all respects except what it does to the body. It attacks and ulcerates intestinal tissue in a random pattern. Weak spots can appear simultaneously from one end of the digestive tract to the other: from the esophagus to the anus, though the vast majority of Crohn's occurs in either intestine. There is no known cause and no known cure, but medication and diet will help put the disease in remission. Diagnosis is touchy, because Crohn's sneaks up slowly, and because the symptoms suggest other diseases. My own symptoms would remain with me, mostly in lessening stages, for a year. And I would be on medication for four years.

After nearly two months in the hospital on IV's, which I rolled into the bathroom with me many times each day, I went home weighing 86 pounds. I struggled to get the mental picture together, to say: "Well, I'm not a freak after all. They found out what it is." I still felt like a freak.

The first two weeks out of the hospital were a running nightmare that worsened each night. Despite my frail body I perceived myself to be a 1,000-pound stone around my parents' necks. Mom and Dad, who mistakenly thought of Crohn's as being something like an ulcer, falsely blamed each other for causing it. Dad said Mom had stomach problems, and had passed them on to me. Mom said Dad's late-night arrivals from a night at the bar —after which they would argue—made me nervous. And I, of course, blamed myself for causing *their* bickering. Now we were truly a dysfunctional family.

Tension and stress do not cause Crohn's. But when stress is introduced to an existing Crohn's situation, it's the icing on an ugly cake. Think of yourself in the most messed-up gastro situation you have ever experienced—be it flu or whatever. Then imagine putting yourself under the most stress you've ever experienced. *Now* imagine what's going on in your abdomen. So it went on Sixty-Seventh Street, in spades.

I suspect that everyone, once or twice in their life, considers choosing not to live anymore. For teenagers, who haven't had the pain and privilege of seeing their way through serious adversities, the lure of suicide is amplified a hundred times. Even minor obstacles seem overwhelming. My obstacle was that I was living in a body torn up in ways I couldn't have imagined—except maybe in a 90-year-old. I was loaded with physical and emotional scar tissue, 99 percent of it on the inside.

If anybody ever had more self-pity, he's the champ. I wanted people to suck up to me, to take care of me. And they did. Some of the neighborhood people laughed at her, but Mom kept delivering the Daily News for me—in the snow—so I wouldn't lose the job. I couldn't go to school, so the school sent tutors to the house. I wanted people to be sympathetic, and I played every ace in the deck to make it happen.

But was this the way I had to live—with my mother babying

me and going out of her way to prepare just the right foods and my father, when he did get home to dinner, saying, "Oh, we have to have *this* again?" And me running out of the room? I began to think, "Let's get the razor blade out, because I'm just a hassle to everybody."

One night at the dinner table I took a dish of food—I can't remember what it was, except that it was steaming hot—and threw it against a wall, shattering the plate and leaving a gooey trail down to the floor.

There was dead silence.

Then everybody started crying. And then babbling. What's going on here? Let's regroup!

It was a good talk. For my part, I realized that all this self-pity wasn't me. It was an act. And once again I tried to get my mental program in gear. When it happened, it was near-instantaneous. If you drew a graph of it, you would see a long curve sinking to the bottom of the page—and then a vertical line going almost straight north out of sight. Really. That's the way it played out.

After our talk, I realized that Mom and Dad were going to lead a happily married life again, despite this little obstacle who lived in the next room. I realized that the school would function without me. I realized that street hockey had not disappeared from Brooklyn in my absence. I realized that it wasn't any fun being sick. I wanted to do something about it.

Once I broke through the self-pity, everything Dr. Imperato had told me suddenly made sense. It was illuminated on a neon billboard a mile high. I could go into a corner and melt away and cease to exist; or I could take this handicap and turn it into a challenge. It wasn't the world against me. It was ME AGAINST ME.

I can't really begin to explain what happened at the moment that billboard lit up, except that it *was* a moment, it was mid-January 1977, it wasn't daylight yet, and I know exactly what I did next. I got in my 1970 red Maverick and drove down to the waterfront. Not to take my life, but to *celebrate* it.

At the west end of Brooklyn, the Verazanno Narrows Bridge hangs across the sky. If the hard hats who create these blue-collar works of art ever once understood what they were doing—besides stringing massive coils of steel, driving rivets and making welds—this must be the once. It's the world's longest suspension bridge, a hard-hat masterpiece running from Brooklyn to Staten Island.

When I was five years old, my Dad would take me down to the water to fly a kite. The bridge towers were already up, but that summer we watched them hang the deck. It was a picture I would never forget. As years went by, it became my personal reality check. If you ever get to Brooklyn, you've got to see it for yourself. Brooklyn isn't exactly a tourist destination, but you're not going to beat this view anywhere.

Put yourself on the Brooklyn shore of the narrows, just above the bridge. Turn your head from right to left and you'll see the whole world go by.

Up the Hudson River lies the southern tip of Manhattan, the clutter capital of the world, 26 miles of skyscrapers and glitz and poverty and geniuses and crazy people. Then your eyes come down to the Statue of Liberty—out in the water where the Hudson River and the East River come together—with various incidentals in the background, like New Jersey. Then, as you pan to the left, comes Staten Island and this awesome bridge skying over to it. Beyond the bridge you see nothing and everything—*forever*, the Lower Bay and on out into the Atlantic Ocean. In one wink you go from seeing this incredible concentrated mass of people and money, to seeing infinity where no one walks.

I love water. I love sunrises. I can't count the times I rode my bicycle down to look at the water, look at the bridge, look at the high-rises.

Shore Road runs along the water, and above it lie the high-rises of the Bay Ridge neighborhood. These apartments mesmerized me nearly as much as the bridge. This was the elite section of Brooklyn. The view was a lot different than from Sixty-Seventh Street, three blocks from where *Saturday Night Fever* was shot at the Club 2001 Odyssey. A few months later in '77, the whole country would be watching John Travolta and his Bensonhurst pals being drawn to the bridge.

On that crisp January morning I took a blanket, got in the Maverick, drove down to Shore Road and waited for the sun to come up.

It must have been about 17 degrees. I parked on a hill going down to the Beltway and shivered under my blanket and watched the cars going by, and then watched the dawn rise left to right across water and the bridge and the Statue of Liberty. You're getting the picture already and it's just too corny, but it is absolutely 100 percent the way it was. I thought about what an asshole—to use an ironic, profane and accurate word—I had been. And I said to myself, "Damn. I want to live. I want to *live*."

Some kind of fire was lit that morning. It was as if all the internalizing, all the negativism, all the pain and hurt, all the fear had been constricted for so long and now were let loose from a catapult. I was sitting still in the old Maverick but I was moving forward at the speed of light.

I wanted to thank everybody—from Mom who delivered the papers to the docs who carved me up, even if the system did treat you like a dog. I wanted to thank the school for sending tutors. I wanted to thank my Dad for showing me this bridge. It was like an Academy Award acceptance speech run amok. I thanked people who would have been stone shocked if they had heard the thanks.

I thanked God, of course. And I struck a deal. This wasn't really a prayer. It wasn't really even in a religious mode, it was more like the cliche of the guy hanging from a cliff or going underwater for the last time who suddenly starts thinking real hard about the deity. Anyway, I struck a deal.

I told the Man Upstairs that if He would just make me better, I would do *anything*. Make me normal and I will not get in trouble on street corners, I will not take so many things for granted, I will listen to the doctor, I will take care of myself, I will make *myself* healthy, I *will not be this cocky kid from Brooklyn*. And on and on.

It was a powerful fire that was lit out there on Shore Road. Because everything that has happened to me since then I can trace to that moment.

I wouldn't blame you if you said a Hollywood scriptwriter wouldn't dream up that story. In fact, when *Rocky II* got to the neighborhood I said to myself: "You know, I had more going against me than he did."

4

"They Look Like Toothpicks"

When the surgeons were through cutting, Dr. Imperato told my parents to put me on a nutritious diet and to avoid milk products because of my lactose intolerance. And, oh yeah, this kid has to get his body back—so you ought to get him a 110-pound set of weights.

My father went out and bought a set as a belated Christmas present. It was sitting in the basement the morning I went down to the waterfront. Those weights were among the 56 million things I thought about as the sun came up. And I thought about them in ways I never had before.

About a year earlier, my cousin, Louis Romanzi, had taken me to Boston College for a visit. Louis played football at BC, and this was my first chance to schmooze with some big-time athletes. I was impressed. When I saw all these guys in the weight room pumping iron, I thought, yeah, it would be nice to build your body into something that awesome. But I didn't feel the least inclined to put in that kind of sweat, that much work. It never occurred to me that bodybuilding would ever be a part of my life.

Louis wasn't just an iron-pumping football player, he was a genuine bodybuilder. When I'd visit my uncle's house in Bayshore, I'd pick up some of Louis's muscle magazines. And I'd laugh at the whole idea. This was a sport? And I'd say something to Louis like: "These guys are all either gay or they're muscleheads." Which was pretty bold, considering that Louis was older and at least 100 pounds heavier. I remember looking at a picture of Arnold Schwarzenegger all greased up, and I said: "Why would anybody want to do that to their body?" I couldn't comprehend what it was all about.

But when my last semester started at Fort Hamilton, I signed up for weight training. It was only once a week, though, and I didn't work very hard. I probably missed a few of the sessions because of illness before I left school for good and went into the hospital. I learned how to tell a barbell from a dumbbell, and a curl from a press. That was the extent of my weightlifting knowledge on January 17, 1977.

I can't forget that date. I've become a goal-oriented person, and I write my goals down on paper. When a day goes badly, or if something gives me even a trace of self-pity, I open up a kitchen cabinet and there it is: a calendar with all my goals for the year—including the ones I've already achieved, neatly checked off. Try it; you'll be surprised what it will do for your perspective and focus. The very first date I ever wrote down was January 17, 1977. I was in the basement of our apartment building, and I decided to log my progress as I built my body back to what I dreamed of being above all else: *normal.*

The doctors at the hospital had said not to exercise for a month. But the fire was lit and I was ready. Well, actually, my physical strength was more like an ember than a fire; but the fire in my mind *was* ablaze. I was careful. Just a few curls and a couple of bench presses at a time. I didn't do sit-ups because of the bag on my stomach.

Despite my light little effort at exercise, my mother and grandmother would come rushing down the stairs to make sure I wasn't hurting myself. I had made these great strides forward and didn't need any more babying, but I was getting it anyway. There was a big difference. Now it was comical instead of tragic.

I turned my life around down that 100-year-old basement. That's serious. But there was a slapstick element to it all.

For starters, I could only make a space about eight feet wide. And the ceiling was low—about six feet—which meant you couldn't do any work standing up. There was dust all over the place, which didn't help my various allergies. The smell was atrocious—first because of your own sweat in a cramped and airless space, and then because I was right next to the garbage pails and the incinerator chute. I'd be counting reps, and on "six" a dead fish or such would hit bottom a couple of feet away. On the other side of the "gym" were the clotheslines, usually loaded with sheets and underwear. And you always had people walking through, going to the clotheslines or to the garbage cans.

Welcome to the Original Peter Nielsen's Eye of the Tiger Total Fitness Club. I should have had business cards printed up. Down at the bottom they'd proclaim: "Unmatched Ambience."

About two months after coming home from the hospital, I went back. The doctors took the bag came off my stomach. I cannot tell you what it meant to a 15-year-old for this particular roll of the dice to come up a winner. It meant, most basically, that on my 16th birthday—March 16, 1977—I would be performing a basic bodily function normally, the way I assumed every other 16-year-old in the universe performed it. Clearly, somebody was answering those promises I made on Shore Road. In later years, speaking around the country to raise money for research into Crohn's and other bowel diseases, I would come into contact with scores of people who are leading normal, productive, happy lives without the luxury of reversing that roll of the dice. It's just one of the thousands of ways I have learned that whatever your circumstance, others have it worse. And whatever you achieve, others have done more.

Fueled by my new degree of freedom, I became even more of a terror with my 110-pound set of weights. I added another few iron plates and picked up some dumbbells. By the time I was finished with my grandmother's basement, I probably had a thousand dollars worth of equipment down there.

These were fun times. The tutors came to the apartment, and in the end I graduated six months ahead of everybody else. I basically had nothing to do but study and bring my body back. I started alone, and then Frankie Puccio—my hockey-playing friend from across the hall—joined me. And then Tommy Lupo from Sixty-Fourth Street. We were three oddball musketeers, pumping iron amid the fish carcasses and the drying underwear from 3C. One time one of us pushed some iron a little too high and snapped a plumbing pipe. Now we had the only gym in town with a water hazard.

In the beginning I worked with a little supermarket book that showed how to do different exercises. Then I started to wonder about this whole *bodybuilding* thing. I had to be impressed with Lou Ferrigno. He was almost from the neighborhood, growing up two miles away on Sixty-Fourth Street, and he was a Mr. Universe—soon to be immortalized as *The Incredible Hulk*, the green guy with all those muscles. I kept buying exercise books, learning new material like a sponge.

I learned so much down that basement, not just about working out, but about life and reality. Years later I would own a gym with half a million dollars worth of equipment in it. But to this day I work out wearing my father's old telephone lineman's belt. It works just fine. I don't care what brand name is on the tags of your sweats or on the heel of your shoes. They can all be ragged, and that's fine with me. Fancy gloves? I've got calluses, not gloves. Never once as the years went on did I get impressed or taken in by pricey paraphernalia, because it didn't mean a thing in my basement gym. All that mattered was the *fire*. If you've got it—my version of it or your version of it—nothing else matters.

We improvised like jazz musicians. We took what was there and made it into something better. Bricks? The basement was full of them. I'd use bricks as a platform for back exercises, or I'd place them so my feet would have more of a stretch when I lay down. Outside in the courtyard, when the weather got warmer, I'd use the fence gate as a brace for dips. I'd hold on to a tree for stretch exercises. I did pull-ups on a tree branch.

The point is, not having a fancy health club membership is no excuse if you want to work out. If you can't afford it, or if you just don't want to work out in public, no problem. Do you have a *chair* in your house? A rope? A towel? All these things can be excellent pieces of exercise equipment when you are creative.

In the basement, my self-education pursued an exercise curriculum. Upstairs in the apartment I was launching my education in nutrition. To begin with, I made myself a human guinea pig.

Let's see, today's subject is lactose intolerance. Let's try some pizza. OK, stomach all torn up, off to the bathroom. Experiment complete. Thesis confirmed: You play, you pay.

I had to learn big-time. The doctors saved my life, but nutrition was not their specialty. And the mystery of Crohn's, particularly in a teenaged patient, had them beating a path to *my* lab. I'd get a call. "Peter, what happened when you had that binge and ate two slices of pizza?" And I'd say: "Well, doctor, the first two slices weren't bad . . ." And somebody would document the bad news.

I took vitamins and I tried protein powders. I read everything I could find on the subject. The real dietary tricks of preparing for a bodybuilding competition would come later. But very quickly I found myself well-versed in basic, sound nutrition. I learned what proteins and carbohydrates and fats mean to your body, where they go and what they do when they get there. I put myself on a dietary regimen that at first was merely an exercise in discipline, but which I soon learned was an exercise in health. In other words, I started to feel better.

All in all, the self-pitying kid who had wanted to strike out at a very wise doctor was coming out of his shell. These were exciting times.

These were also scary times.

Not long after leaving the hospital, my blood count was still wrong. The mono had returned. I had to fight that off.

Then, about a month after having the bag removed, I returned to the hospital for a scope test that would check all of the repair work on my plumbing. The doctors found cancerous polyps on my colon, totally unrelated to the Crohn's. The polyps were tiny, and the doctors scraped them off with no trouble. But they were cancer. And they scared the hell out of me.

I'm not sure what would have happened if I had heard the word "malignant" when I was in the hospital at Christmastime. Two months later, it was no picnic. But I had set out on my way along my little obstacle course with a completely different head on my shoulders. A new head, and working toward a new body. Not many days after the doctors scraped away the polyps, I was back down among the garbage pails pumping iron.

I reached a healthy plateau down there with my slowly growing collection of weights—and my radio. Music was always important to me. I played lead guitar and sang in a neighborhood garage band that we put together back in the sixth grade. Our first public appearance was at a block party where we conned the hired band into letting us sit in for one song. These four rockin' little kids upstaged the older guys, and a career of sorts was launched. We played Bensonhurst parties and weddings for almost a decade. My sister joined the band, playing tambourine and singing. I always wondered if, in another roll of the dice, I might have had a career as a singer. Probably not; that series of broken noses made my intonation pretty nasal.

The music on my radio was background to a steady, pleasant groove: Work out in the basement, meet with the tutors, study, work out in the basement, pore over anything I could find to read about nutrition and exercise, experiment in the kitchen, work out in the basement.

I had never before known what it was like to feel good. The Crohn's had always been there, just waiting to come full-blown out of remission. That happened when I was 15. It could have happened when I was six, or 60. But from toddling age onward I had been a sickly kid. I was a short kid because I wasn't getting proper nourishment. Every birthday I would get fever and chills because anxiety—even though it doesn't *cause* Crohn's—can work with the disease to trigger gastro problems. So I was a thin, short, quick-to-tire kid who got sick whenever something made him nervous. My parents say that whole syndrome started back when I was three. Finally getting well and putting some musculature on my body was an indescribable high.

In January 1978, a year and a month after my Crohn's surgery, I became a certified mid-year home-tutored graduate of Fort Hamilton High School. I was well on the way to putting my disease into remission, still the proud owner of a 1970 Maverick, and no longer looking anorexic. By mid-summer of 1978 I was probably a whopping 145 pounds or so. I felt like Hercules.

It was never my intention to set foot in a real gym. But all the magazines said that if you wanted to make genuine progress, you had to be in a competitive environment, had to have somebody a little better pushing you ahead.

Meantime, a friend of my mother's told me about a guy in Flatbush. He trains champions, she said. You ought to check him out, she said.

So I did.

The guy in Flatbush was Julie Levine, chiropractor by trade, powerlifter by avocation. When I walked in his door he stood about 5-foot-10, half an inch shorter than me, and carried a very compact 200 pounds or so.

His place was R&J Health Studios on Avenue U between East Twenty-Seventh and East Twenty-Eighth streets. This was the East Coast Mecca of bodybuilding. I didn't understand the first thing about that. I just knew this was where Lou Ferrigno had trained, and that Julie had been Ferrigno's manager, and that if you didn't know about Ferrigno at that time, then you probably weren't alive—and you definitely weren't in Brooklyn. But I didn't know the first thing about Julie.

I introduced myself and Julie said: "Hi ya kid, howya doin'? Looks like ya been trainin' your arms a couple years. What happened to your legs? They look like toothpicks."

Helloooo, Julie. Welcome to the gym.

Devastated. Hurt. Embarrassed for my basement gym and the bricks and the garbage cans and . . . what was this runt—me—doing here anyway?

But you know what? Adversity really *had* become my best friend. The bad vibes lasted maybe 30 seconds. Then Julie's little insult bounced off me and I got on with business.

Under my breath I called Julie every profane name I knew. And then I paid him $178 for a year's membership. In a long and strong relationship, it was the only time Julie ever charged me for using R&J's facilities.

Mecca of Bodybuilders or not, moving up to Julie's was not like moving from the basement to some plush-carpeted suburban health spa. At R&J, if you didn't smell the sweat, you had pneumonia. The place was very famous but not very swank. It had characters and character. My ragged attire fit right in.

Walking down the stairs you had to watch yourself, because pieces of the steps were missing. The dumbbells were the big old round type, with chips knocked out by too many collisions with the floor. You'd have to calibrate: Let's see, this is an 85-pounder, but with that chunk gone it's probably about 79.

This wasn't a wealthy section of Brooklyn, and neither was there any facade on anybody who pumped iron at R&J. The customers—ranging in age from the teens to the 70s—just wanted to be the best that they could be. Basically they were vulgar, full of lies about their romantic conquests of the previous evening, and not real interested in where the Dow Jones Average was going this afternoon. It was a social club with the aroma of exercise. It was wonderful.

Julie presided like a revered bartender. R&J wasn't a health *salon,* it was a health *saloon*—like a good neighborhood bar you'd start hanging out in at 20 and stay until you died, as long as that same guy was standing there with the towel and the talk. If he dies, the bar dies.

Seventeen years old, training at Julie's place, surrounded by bodybuilders, full of myself because my body and I had fought the Crohn's into remission—no way do you get this far down the road without checking out what lies around the bend. So I slipped out of town to enter my first bodybuilding contest. It was Mr. Armstrong County, a teenaged amateur competition somewhere in Pennsylvania. My father drove eight hours to get us there. I finished fifth.

I remember sleeping in the back seat with my trophy. And I remember seeing the face of the person who won, and I knew that this was something I really wanted to do—at least to finish first one time. If I was going to do it, R&J would be the place where it would come together. I had made it 90 percent of the way down in Grandma's basement, but the very tough remaining 10 percent needed Julie and the gym.

First I went to work on my "toothpicks." At home I was zeroing in on nutrition. At Julie's I was zeroing in on my legs, working to show this wiseguy what I could do. I added nine inches to my thighs.

In my next competition, Mr. Teenage Appalachia, I won my class and finished second overall. But one judge said I looked like a freak. My legs were too big.

5

Trophy Time

That chilly sunrise monologue out on Shore Road lingered in my mind like deathbed testimony. I was on trial, having promised the moon in return for becoming a normal kid. So I became a gym rat with all the dedication of an avowed monk. Julie's gym, however, was a different sort of monastery. And cloistering was not a part of the vows.

I began to fantasize how far I might get in this newly discovered world of bodybuilding. It was an irresistible quantum leap—from a kid whose body had nearly rotted him to death before he was old enough for a regular driver's license, to a Danish/Italian Adonis from Brooklyn. Why not? Ferrigno got his start at Julie's. Someday, I said to myself a couple of times when I was sure no mind readers were nearby, they'll say: This is where Peter Nielsen worked out.

Nobody worked harder.

Julie learned a lot about me from the way I responded to his wisecrack about my legs. "You can't say things like that to certain people," Julie said. "But I knew you could take it." He didn't know any such thing, of course. He was just lucky he stumbled onto somebody for whom turning negatives into positives had become a specialty. And I was just lucky that I stumbled onto Julie.

It also turned out I was lucky to have had those karate lessons I hated so much. I had dreaded the ride to Flatbush every single time my Dad took me to class. Karate wasn't in my heart. I think I earned my brown belt just because of all the animosity I built up on the ride over. By the time I got there, I'd want to crush everybody in the place because I despised being there so much. Let's get this over with! Uuhhhhhh! Take that.

But karate introduced me to discipline and self-esteem. It taught me how to choreograph my body, to have better timing. It really gave me confidence—even with the opposite sex, with dancing, being more agile. And by the time I got into bodybuilding competition, those dreaded old karate sessions helped me with my posing the same way ballet lessons had helped Schwarzenegger. There is a macho side to all this that no man can understand until, first, he achieves a body that can handle it, and second, he tries it. When you take that body up on stage not to recite a few choice words, not to play a piano, not to dunk a basketball, but to display for a few moments the distillation of hundreds of hours of athletic sweat—*that* is a supreme confidence check. It involves guts and it involves grace.

Almost from the beginning, I had an affinity for posing. It's a major part of competition. If you want to win, you can't look like you'd rather be somewhere else. Something about the pain and scars of my illness made me thrive on the soul-baring that goes with being up on stage all alone. It's not how well you swing a bat, or how much gold you're wearing around your neck —*you* are the product. Whatever you have done with what God has given you, and with your wisdom and sweat and proper eating habits, this is your way of showing how good you can be as a person on the physical level. Maybe it was because my physical being had dwindled almost to nothing that putting its reconstructed polar opposite on display seemed such a natural step; I don't know.

I do know that striking a pose—coming "cut," as they say when a competitor brings muscles to their full definition—means meeting insecurity head-on. You had better be ready, physically and mentally, or you are going to crash like an SST nosing into a rock. And I know that, for me, there was a pride and a freedom and a sense of achievement like I had never experienced before.

Julie put me on track. In 1979 he first got me posing in front of a mirror almost every day, showing me how to check out my body parts, how to tailor an exercise regimen that would take me toward symmetry. He made me see self-examination as part of the craft. You win or you lose because of what the judges see. If you want to improve what they see, then you've got to learn how to evaluate for yourself what all those bench presses and curls and dips are producing on your body, and where to make adjustments.

We started taking all this seriously not long after the Teenage Apppalachia contest—it seemed like they were always far away. Dad drove me to all of them. In 1979, I became a teenaged terror, winning one contest after another. Once I won two contests in a single weekend. My training was together, my diet was together, and it was all paying off.

And there was a girl, wise beyond her years, named Yvonne Wind. Even today when I hear Bette Midler singing *You Are the Wind Beneath My Wings* I think of Yvonne. She lived near the gym, taking care of her emphysematic father, and we started dating soon after I first met Julie. Sunrise promises on Shore Road or not, I'm not sure I would have taken this bodybuilding thing so far without Yvonne.

She'd cook dinner for me, make sure I got over to Julie's even if I wasn't in the mood, sit down and learn nutrition with me, encourage me. Even cocky street kids thrive on encouragement. After I won my first contest, Yvonne made it seem like I was on the cover of *Sports Illustrated* when I really wasn't anywhere except on Julie's bulletin board. This was a teenaged romance that meant something.

My Dad—who at first regarded bodybuilding as weirdness from deep leftfield—began to see that it was good for me. He even got caught up a little in the competitiveness. When the weekend came, we'd hop in the car and go pick up another trophy. But a total, full-time commitment to the sport was something else. To Dad, that was still *deep* leftfield.

And I was totally committed. Except for making a few bucks doing odd-job construction, my only work was on my body and my mind. Both kept getting stronger, and the trophies started piling up. By standard measurements of success, however, I had become your basic well-proportioned dropout.

In 1980, when I was still 19, Dad cut a lot of red tape and wined and dined his boss to get me my first and only "legitimate" nine-to-five job—as a lineman's assistant for New York Bell, following in his footsteps, making decent money, enjoying full health-care coverage. This was the real world, and this was a job to be prized. The streets were full of people who would kill for a job as a lineman's assistant.

The first doorbell I rang was to make a disconnect, for non-payment, in Bedford-Stuyvesant. A heavyset woman with a serious attitude answered the door, and people started screaming in the hallway. I put my screwdriver up to remove a phone jack and a gang of roaches came crawling out of the wall. Then a very large man emerged from a bedroom and joined in the shouting. Out back, where I had to disconnect and test some other wires, a group of very tough-looking guys were playing cards. I did my job and got in the truck.

"You wanna know something?" I told my partner. "*No* amount of money is worth this."

Ten days later, I quit. I went to my boss and told him I was sorry. He said, "Don't worry. Your Dad is going to take this a lot worse than I am."

He was right.

Dad couldn't understand the dreams that were forming in my mind. All he knew was that I had come out of the hospital three years earlier as a sick kid and was doing OK—but devoting all my time to lifting weights and counting grams of protein and fat. And now I was spitting on a job that he had used to raise a son and a daughter. All he saw in the gym was ego. He didn't fully understand the will to survive that had led me to the gym. He didn't understand at all my discovery that pumping iron might lead me to a world of achievement. For my part, I was a few years away from the maturity to understand the difference between making something an important *part* of your life and making it your *whole* life. I guess this was your classic clash of the generations.

Anyway, my father quit talking to me.

By now, Julie Levine realized that this kid from Bensonhurst possessed a level of determination that went somewhere far beyond the ordinary. He devoted still more time to my physical program, and to jawing with me about what it takes to be a champion. I was on track for the Eastern Teenage America, by far my most serious competition yet, and Julie was getting on track with me.

That's when I knew I had the opportunity of a lifetime. I was learning everything from gym etiquette to kinesiology from the master himself. One thing Julie preached was not to take things too seriously, not to lose perspective. I was young. Some of Julie's lessons I absorbed better than others.

One day Julie took me to see a doctor of sports medicine who worked with bodybuilders. He gave Julie an honest assessment, the way a horse trainer might analyze the conformation of a thoroughbred. Not while I was in the room, of course.

Genetics can give a bodybuilder a handicap or a head start. Just as you won't see too many six-foot-10 and 290-pound figure skaters, you won't see champion body builders with ultra-high calves or biceps, or with long legs beneath a short torso. This is the sort of thing the sports doctor was evaluating for Julie.

A few weeks later I got the message secondhand when I overheard Julie talking to somebody else. The doc's diagnosis? Peter will become a local champion, possibly a state champion. If he's tremendously lucky, he'll become a regional champion. As far as a national champion, I'd put my license against it.

More wood for the fire! If negatives were the raw material I used to build my positive outlook, I was definitely a rich kid. I'm sure Julie didn't intend for me to hear that conversation, but it was a good thing I did. You can lift a lot of barbells and skip a lot of junk food with words like that ringing in your ears.

All of these teenaged contests were amateur events. The Eastern America show was big-time nonetheless. It was at Lincoln Center, and it seemed like half of Brooklyn made the trip into Manhattan. My Mom was there, Julie was there, half of his clientele was there, and if things got dull we could have put my old street hockey team together in 30 seconds.

If you've ever seen a bodybuilding competition, you know the finals don't get dull. Most of the serious judging is done in the afternoon, away from the crowds, the same as compulsories in figure skating. The afternoon scene can be like going into a college gym and stumbling onto a hard-fought game in some minor sport. The players and officials are intent, all right, but not much is happening otherwise. Then at night, when the finals of a bodybuilding competition occur, the scene changes dramatically.

There's a crowd, there's music, there are spotlights, there is an exuberant emcee. Every contestant has a claque, his own followers, cheering wildly for or against each competitor. If a bodybuilder happens to be from Brooklyn, the cheering is likely to be more colorful than if he is from, say, White Plains. And when you do your posing in front of that crowd, you are a very long way from the solitude of a mirror at R&J Health Studios.

Lincoln Center was also a long way from Pennsylvania and New Jersey and some of the other outposts where Dad had taken me to win various local competitions. This uptown contest was wild and scary, and I loved it. I won my height classification, I won best in every body part, I won overall. I wish I had a transcript of what the announcer read that night, with all my Bensonhurst friends stomping and whistling, but I don't. He said something about a young man who had overcome adversity and was on his way up the ladder, and he said: "We have a special presenter to give Peter his trophy as Mr. Eastern Teenage America—Pete Nielsen, Peter's father."

Whatever this thing was that his kid had gotten into, Dad had decided that it must be important. I wasn't an opera singer or an actor or a politician, but I was on the stage of Lincoln Center collecting a trophy. And my father, who hadn't talked to me in six weeks, was handing it to me.

We both got teary-eyed. And Dad was with me for the rest of the run to the top.

He started carrying my posed picture in his wallet, and a glossy of me went up on the wall at the Avenue U Bar. Dad also forgave me for dumping the lineman's assistant job and helped get me put on call for construction work, mainly handling a jackhammer on road crews. Julie canceled my membership fee at R&J and gave me a key so I could work out at 4 a.m. or midnight or whenever it fit my schedule. Life became a crazy pattern of tooth-rattling jackhammer work on weekdays and competitions on weekends. I wore a hard hat and I wore a bikini, I worked under traffic lights and I worked under stage lights, I crunched pavement and I consumed protein. It was an interesting mix. I'm probably the only human being who ever passed through the late teen years and into young adulthood along quite the same career path.

The construction crews usually decided I wasn't wrapped too tight. I was the only construction worker, for instance, who ordered vegetable omelettes made with no yokes. If you're not used to them, egg-white omelettes do look pale. On the other hand, it's the cholesterol and fat that you're leaving in the kitchen.

Then one day I did a number on a taxi driver and my construction crew colleagues became convinced the kid was truly weird. It seems like every time I ever worked on a jackhammer it was either 100 degrees in the shade or minus-10. On the day in question it was so cold I was shaking *before* I picked up my hammer. I worked under this little framed tent that was supposed to keep the wind chill off me, and I was rattling and hammering and chipping and shivering right in the center lane. The cabbie pulled up, laid on his horn, sat there and kept braying away. Only a New York cab driver would sit in traffic and honk his horn at a tent.

I was cold and miserable and this honking was a genuine irritation. In a second, the cabbie wasn't irritated—he was so scared he nearly relieved himself in the fare box. My body was in pretty good shape by then, so I cradled this 70-pound jackhammer like it was an Uzi, raised my left arm in the air like I was leading a charge on enemy lines, and came running out of the tent pulling the trigger. The cabbie must have thought he'd stumbled onto Rambo dressed for the Russian front. He stopped blowing his horn. My co-workers just rolled their eyes.

One morning about 4 a.m. I was going into R&J and had just put the key in the door when a guy came walking out of the restaurant next door, saying goodbye to everybody. He couldn't have been more than six feet away. A car pulled up to the curb and all of a sudden - pow, pow, pow—the guy next to me falls to the sidewalk with parts of his head missing. The car pulled slowly away.

Like I said, it was an interesting life-style for a teenager.

In suburbia, or in farm country, or in small-town middle America—or maybe even in most of urban America—a bodybuilder can more or less disappear into the woodwork. Most Americans either live far apart, or they get up in the morning and zip from their garage to their office like a deposit slip zooming to the teller at a drive-in bank. If somebody has a little musculature on his body, it either disappears into his work clothes or into the cocoon where he eats and sleeps. Bensonhurst and Flatbush were something else.

Everybody crammed together and nobody hiding. The streets full of people. Life fast-paced and *a la carte*. When I moved to Michigan and somebody picked up a phone and said, "Let's get a pizza," it was the funniest thing I ever heard. Nobody gets a pizza. You get a *slice* of pizza. And you fold it and eat on the run, whether you're wearing rags or a three-piece suit. When I was a kid in Brooklyn, you bought your slice at the pizza parlor. You wanted bread, you went to the bakery. But if you wanted bagels, you went to the bagel shop. It was *a la carte*—a different store for everything.

I had a friend who worked at a *pork* shop. Five zillion cuts of meat and sausages, but not an ounce of beef or chicken or fish in sight. My friend once said, "Peter, I'm working out but I'm still flabby." And I told him, "I think you ought to find a new job."

With everybody out on the street, playing hockey or hustling a buck or getting to work or running between the bakery and the pork shop, Brooklyn was just as different from suburbia as it was from a farm in Kansas. On a hot summer day, strolling down the sidewalk wearing a T-shirt, anybody who spent a lot of time in the gym stood out like a red popcorn kernel in a bag of white.

Somebody who was a cool macho dude was a "coozhine" (say coo-ZHEEN). John Travolta's character in *Saturday Night Fever* was a coozhine. It's a look, an attitude. And bodybuilding was most definitely a good way to be a coozhine in Brooklyn.

I don't mean to overstate this, but there's more of a bodybuilding tradition, history—culture—in some places than others. It's like jazz musicians. Why are such an overwhelming percentage of the truly great jazz players black? Well, that's a complicated question. But one reason is that a lot of black musicians grew up in a culture that attached some importance to the music, gave it some respect. If you wanted to go down your basement and play scales for 10 hours a day, that was OK, because that's what it takes to become a truly great jazz musician. That's the musician's sweat equity. Sometimes you'd have a basement, or a neighborhood, that produced an amazing number of great jazz musicians. Among bodybuilders, Brooklyn was such a neighborhood. And R&J was the best basement of all.

I kept the promises I made, and my body was responding. I was healthy. I was also collecting more trophies than anybody. It was fun being a coozhine.

6

Muscle Glitz

I dreamed of having my own apartment in Bay Ridge, overlooking the narrows and that incredible panorama from Manhattan to infinity. Mom and Dad were supportive. Needless to say, my sister was supportive. My freedom would mean freedom for her in our tiny apartment.

My parents told me: Save up before you move up; get yourself a job and sign a lease. My response? Hey; I've got a month's rent. I've got a security deposit. I'm goal-oriented. Who cares if I don't have a regular job?

I'm not sure it occurred to me that I also didn't have any furniture.

I knew just the place I wanted. I moved in shortly after flunking out as a telephone lineman's assistant. I wrestled the jackhammer and made the rent. But I still spent a lot of time on Sixty-Seventh Street, because some of the finest Italian cooking you'll ever find was still upstairs in my Mom's kitchen.

At night, though, I rested my head in Bay Ridge. I could do my running along Shore Road. I had an *elite* address. The sunrise was free every day, and the water and the bridge came with it.

It was September 1980, and I was 19. From then through the fall of 1984 I would win another 60 bodybuilding trophies. I would suffer two serious relapses of Crohn's. I would pose in Times Square and have my picture in *Newsweek* and the *National Enquirer* and I would appear on *Good Morning, America*. I would go to Central America to win my biggest title, and I would make personal appearances on several continents. I would make some decent money. I'm very proud of those achievements, but the picture was never quite as rosy as it should have been.

For one thing, I was surrounded by dry rot in the form of anabolic steroids. In the early '80s I think it would have been fair to lift an eyebrow at nearly any athlete of tremendous bulk and Adonis proportions. In the '88 Olympics, the Ben Johnson saga proved that you didn't have to be a lumbering football lineman type to enhance your performance with the stuff. My sport, bodybuilding, was awash in steroids as I made my way up.

Two statements I can make unequivocally, with God and however many people buy this book as my witnesses:

First, I never used anabolic steroids.

Second, I came so close that I get sick thinking about it.

The juice was everywhere.

There was a kid up the street from me who was using steroids and bragging about it, even showing syringes to his friends. One day he started passing blood in his urine and got rushed to the hospital. I knew another steroid user who dropped dead of a heart attack in the gym, where he was supposed to be getting healthy.

The most insidious part of the steroid epidemic, in fact, was that the biggest pushers were the athletes themselves. They'd play Russian roulette with liver function tests, smiling when they registered way above normal but just below the point where they'd start bleeding internally. One kid told me he would be willing to take steroids even if he knew it would kill him, as long as he could win Mr. Teenage America first. So much sickness was running around wearing the trappings of fitness.

The pressure to try the stuff was immense, particularly in the teenaged years when the mind lacks maturity—and the muscles have trouble achieving size. I know that many competitors regarded me as a candy-ass for not being a user. And I know that many others believed that I *was* a user and was a candy-ass for lying about it.

I also know that just one of the dozens and dozens of times

another weightlifter pushed anabolic steroids on me in the gym, I bought some. Dynabol. It was my first or second year of working out.

I was young and susceptible. But instead of opening the bottle and starting to pop the stuff like candy, I took it home and stashed it in the bathroom. I don't know if wisdom, ethics, common sense—all the things that insist no human being ever ingest steroids—would have prevailed. I like to think so. But in the end, it was two things— my goal-setting nature and Crohn's disease—that assured I did not take the lunatic path.

Remember my calendar? I wrote down for a Monday: "Start Dynabol." Meanwhile, I would think about it. Thanks to the Crohn's, I didn't have to think too long. I started bleeding internally, with no help whatsoever from anabolic steroids.

Whatever portion of the teenaged fantasy about bottled muscles I might or might not have bought into, it disappeared instantly. I nearly screamed aloud: "What *am* I doing?!" I flushed the steroids down the toilet and went into a cold sweat.

Was I so vulnerable that I could forget why I started lifting weights in the first place? How could I so carefully choose and measure the fuel I put in my body at the dinner table, and then even think about gulping this poison? The stuff isn't even a narcotic, and its pull is that strong. Incredible.

Later, I would go on stage in competitions and discover that the guy on my left and the guy on my right were both pumping steroids as well as iron. I would discover that some bodybuilders I had thought to be natural, were not. A frustrating, contradictory, mentally debilitating knowledge revealed itself over the next four years: Bodybuilding is a great sport that should earn much wider participation and media interest, but—in the form I was seeing every weekend—it was hopelessly corrupted by this deadly genie in a drug bottle.

Today I spend a fair amount of time talking to kids about the danger of drugs—any kind of drugs. I hope my talks do some good. I hold my body up as an example of what they can do "clean and natural" with their own bodies—which is, thank God, 100 percent true. Other people have other ways of trying to get the message across. Whatever works is fine with me. Any "Say no" message is worth the effort. But please, please, don't stick that other word in front of it. *"Just* say no" is the dumbest message on the face of the Earth. If it were a case of *just* saying no, there would be no problem. Whatever things kids do wrong, it isn't because it's the *hard* thing to do. It's because it's the *easy* thing to do.

The other cloud over my rosy four years of glory was in my own head. I kept 100 percent of my Shore Road promises about my body, but it would take a while before I really stopped being that cocky kid from Brooklyn. Glory is a tough thing to handle when you're young. And pretty soon I wasn't just a coozhine—I was *uptown!* I put body-building and the glitz and the glamour ahead of everything and did some incredibly stupid things with my personal life. You might say I suffered creeping muscleheadedness.

I dumped Yvonne, for one thing. And, toward the end of this four-year run, I tried to be a party animal while simultaneously keeping my body in top form. Too many times I met myself in the morning coming from tinseltown to the gym. If you think you can handle that, I'm sorry. It can't be done. Maybe for a quick minute when you're young, and that's it. I was young, and I used my quick minute to the max.

I also spent a lot of money. That's not a sin, and it doesn't affect your training. But it was awfully stupid.

Nonetheless, I have to admit there were times I showed an incredible panache and entrepreneurial spirit for my years.

In 1981, for example, I grew increasingly tired of hanging onto that jackhammer. It seemed to me that if I could spend my weekends striking a pose on stage and collecting all that silverware for my troubles, then there ought to be a way to make a buck at it during the week.

What I did was audacious.

It went something like this: Let's see, this is the greatest country in the world, so I should go into business. What have I got to sell? Well, I've got a physique and some clips from the muscle mags and the *Daily News* and I've got a real talent for posing. Where can I sell that? Well . . . how about Studio 54?

I was like a 20-year-old bomber pilot in World War II. I didn't know I couldn't do it so I did it. I grabbed my portfolio, took off, and dropped it square on the desk of Studio 54's managers.

"Listen," I said pointing to the clips. "This is me. I've won best poser in every single one of my contests."

"Great," said the head man. "So what?"

Well, as I said, music has always been important to me, and I used it in my bodybuilding routine, almost like choreography. But I knew I needed something a little more if I was going to be the first bodybuilder hired to work the country's most famous disco. So I improvised.

"What if I had some smoke? I asked. "Some explosions going off at certain times during the routine? What if I wore a dinner jacket and went through a whole act?"

Mr. 54 was hooked. "Yeah," he said. "Continue."

I could make it much more dramatized than during a competition, where you can't use smoke. I would have some glitter on that dinner jacket, and I'd drink a potion and give the illusion that I was *changing* . . .

And I said, "Well, for that I would usually get $500. But if you hire me two days a week, I'll do it for $300 a shot."

Sold.

The first night was a Thursday, a private party—a birthday bash for Charo, who wound up coochee-coocheeing out of her own cake. But the opening act was Peter Nielsen, Mr. Whatever My Latest Title Was. The music was *Sirus* and *Super Nature*. Suddenly the house lights were gone, the spots came on, all the smoke started rising and I was onstage at Studio 54. It was a major success.

I saw that jackhammer disappearing from my life in the rear-view mirror. But $600 a week wasn't all that much in a very shaky, temporary business—so I went off to talk to the proprietor at Magique.

It was at First Avenue and Sixty-First Street in Manhattan, and it was very much in vogue. Frank Sinatra had a drink or two in the joint. My first approach was to the bouncer, who said: "You gotta be kidding; get to the back of the line."

The next morning I called the owner and pretended to be my own agent—Johnny Giganti or something like that—and got an appointment.

My posing career, about five minutes old, was now bringing in $1,400 a week for three nights' work.

I bought a used Mercedes. I would drop by the family apartment with all this money and Mom would get nervous. She didn't really understand—or maybe didn't believe—where it came from, and I don't blame her. I would ask my father—who figured I would be a dead-broke gym rat when I quit the phone company—"Hey, Dad: You need any cash this week?" I'll never forget when he looked at that first Mercedes (I bought another one later). Dad turned to me and said: "I don't believe it. You're out of control."

Dad was right. But I had to learn the hard way.

There was one positive in this run of glitz that Dad didn't understand, and which would help me find a real life when the run was over. My father thought I was making money with my body, but actually I was making money with my brain. I didn't have the only physique on the Eastern Seaboard. I was just the only one who put it in a package and marketed it to the glamour crowd. I had some vision and some creativity and an entrepreneurial bent.

Julie, my mentor and friend, understood. He had given me all the training and experience I needed. He could have kept me under his wing and had a New York local hero working out of R&J. But, like the true second father that he was, he told me: "Peter, you can do better if you go to Dan Lurie." And he sent me to the man.

Dan is a New York weight-training equipment manufacturer and the publisher of *Muscle Training Illustrated*. As Joe Weider is to the West Coast, Dan Lurie is to the East. He agreed to meet me, saw that I had potential, put me in the centerfold of his magazine, got me on the *Joe Franklin Show* and *Good Morning, America*, had me write a column called "Nielsen's Ratings." Now I wasn't just a kid hyping himself into the spotlight at Studio 54. The exposure Dan got for me was big-time and national.

I had saved up a few bucks from my posing jobs, but with all the publicity Dan generated it got even better. I posed around the country, made a few appearances abroad. I got my second Mercedes. I went to a lot of parties and met celebrities like Kareem Abdul Jabbar and Diana Ross and important people from the long laundry list of connections who sip cocktails and devour expensive snack food on that scene. That, of course, led to more personal appearances.

The jackhammer was long gone. But, in a way, I never escaped that unreal night-and-day flip-flop between two worlds. I still commuted between two incompatible addresses: a world of sweat and nutrition and hard work, and a world of cocktails and hors d'oeuvres and hype. I suppose the American way would have been to sue somebody for whiplash.

What I did was go, on Dan Lurie's money, to Belize, in Central America, and win the 1984-'85 Mr. International Universe. I reaped the cash rewards, began to sink even deeper into the night-and-day morass, and finally realized that my father was absolutely right. I was out of control. And my sport was out of control with steroids.

I had promises to keep. And it was getting difficult. So I announced that I would never compete again as long as I had to square off against bottled bodies.

Get a life, they say. And I did.

7

New Life in Motown

Southeastern Michigan isn't exactly the wilderness. Not with a few million people, urban sprawl, the car companies, major league teams in all four big-time spectator sports and a central city with all the usual problems. It's the fifth-largest TV market, which may be the best way of summing up a town in a couch-potato world. For me, in 1984, Detroit's most important demographic was something it had in common with Pittsburgh and San Francisco and Dallas and Winnemucca, Nevada. *It wasn't New York.* When I had a chance to do a few personal appearances in suburban Detroit, Motown looked like as good a place as any to go into withdrawal from the Big Apple. I was only 23, but it was already eight years since I had dedicated my life—as best as a frightened teenager can dedicate a life—to health. And I wasn't feeling very healthy. I wanted to get away from all the temptations, to get squarely back on track.

My family and friends and familiar turf were in New York; but so were all the things that kept tugging me, as my Dad said, out of control. I had become a creature of excess—too many parties, too many girls, too much sipping Gran Marnier between training sessions, too much time using the weights for recovery instead of for training. I was a kid with his hand constantly in the cookie jar, an overgrown coozhine with his picture in the paper. For me, living in New York was like a drunk pitching his tent outside a distillery.

No offense to my friends and business associates here in Michigan, where I've lived for eight years now, but by comparison Detroit is so laid back that I keep expecting to see the Beach Boys walk by. I've got three phone numbers and an agent and an attorney and an accountant and a beeper and my appointment book gets filled with tiny print. I'm super busy, I've got obligations, I take the usual risks of being an entrepreneur. But that crazy, frantic edge to every minute of every day doesn't exist out here, and I don't miss that part of New York a bit. I'm totally adjusted to my new environment. If I could eat pizza, I'd order a whole pie instead of a slice. And I'd eat it sitting down instead of on the run.

I freed my body in Julie's gym, and I freed my mind in Michigan. Unfortunately, it took more than a change of address. In fact, the early going in Michigan was worse than anything I have ever experienced—except, of course, the Crohn's. That's because I came here with a body by Fisher but with an attitude by Studio 54.

What do you suppose the Brooklyn kid bought to cruise the streets of Motown? Right. Of course. A Porsche 928, black, with several thousand dollars worth of performance extras and a Blaupunkt sound system that put a rock band's bass player right in the passenger seat. The 928 seemed exactly what Mr. International Universe ought to be driving. Coincidentally, the price was almost identical to Mr. International Universe's bank account. My arrival in Detroit was like Dumbo stepping off the circus train.

And what did Mr. International Universe get himself involved in? Right. Of course. A relationship with a woman who enjoyed the good life but wasn't seriously interested in a guy whose income consisted of an occasional personal appearance fee and a small endorsement contract. I might have been a minor celebrity in New York and in the world of bodybuilding, but in Detroit I was lucky to have a part-time gig pitching fruit juice. It was a struggle to put gas in the Porsche, let alone foot the bill for wining and dining a girlfriend who had champagne taste.

I suppose all those Spaniards who came to Middle America looking for gold, only to find buffalo chips and tall grass, must have had a similar reaction. Within a few months, Brooklyn was beckoning, real hard. I could go back to Julie's, where somebody once broke a plate-glass window and took nothing out of the place except one of my posters. (They *were* finally saying, "This is where Peter Nielsen worked out.") I could put on one of my Guinea T's, as they called the tank tops we Italians—even the Danish ones—wore, and I could stroll big-time down Avenue U. No matter how bad things got, I could always run over to Sixty-Seventh Street and get the finest home-made spaghetti dinner in New York. The temptation was huge; not for the glitz, but for the comforts of *home*.

The girlfriend had turned out to be, at least from my own point of view, my most serious relationship since Yvonne. It was more serious, because I was older. But with Yvonne it had been unconditional. This time it wasn't. She was domineering and demanding. She tried to bury me emotionally when I aspired to be more than a boy toy. One day she opened the refrigerator in my apartment and made a statement that changed my life. Really, it did. If you get seriously into this business of changing negatives to positives, you can find inspiration in the damnedest places.

What she said was: "You want a commitment from me? When you can't even make enough money to keep orange juice in the refrigerator?"

She told me I was *just* a bodybuilder, a hunk, that I'd never make it as an entrepreneur, that she spent more cash on clothes in a year than I made in a year, that I ought to go back to Brooklyn and "live happily ever after." In that instant, the very last thing I wanted to do was put on a Guinea T and stroll Avenue U.

If Julie's remark about my "toothpick" legs stoked my fire, this woman was tossing gunpowder into a furnace. I was hurt. To be specific, I got tears in my eyes. But then I did the old negative-to-positive double take. The inner fire was roaring.

"You know something, sweetheart," I said, "I'm going to become *so* successful. You're going to turn on TV and see me. You're going to pick up the newspaper and see me. You're going to see my name in lights so bright that when you go down the road you're going to have to take a detour."

Was this kid from Brooklyn, or what? Walk like a man, talk like a coozhine.

I was insecure, to say the least, but I was determined to make something happen instead of retreating to Brooklyn. I was just 23, however, and this was the real world. The days of Studio 54 and Magique were several years, 700 miles and a bucket of reality away. No quick tricks, no smoke and mirrors.

Every day I went to the gym and left a lot of mental garbage there—just like I always had, another example of how pumping iron is good for a lot more than filling out a T-shirt. I made a few bucks as I developed a personal training clientele, not just with the weights but with nutrition counseling and motivation. I began to understand more fully that if you devote your life to practicing and studying something, you acquire knowledge worth passing on to other people.

In the gym rat world, PT means personal training. In the medical world, it means physical therapy. I also began to understand that I was developing expertise in both versions of PT. I'm not a registered physical therapist, let alone an MD, but since age 15 I've had an obvious special affinity for people who are trying to make frail bodies better, who because of illness or accident or years of sedentary life do not fit your standard stereotype of a gym rat. So I was paying special attention to that part of my PT work, bringing out whatever percentage of improvement can be gained in bodies inflicted by lupus or arthritis, among other diseases. And, since personal training is not something that everybody can afford, I began seeing a lot of the sour fruits of affluence—smart, successful achievers whose lifestyle took care of business but left their bodies flabby and destined for intensive care. My dedication to fitness was expanding outward from my own frame toward helping others. I kept myself in shape, and I walked what I talked nutritionally, but I never gave a thought to the juiced-up world of competitive bodybuilding.

I had plenty of motivation to keep seeking the spotlight in other ways. For one thing, I enjoyed it. Let's face it, when you grow up playing street hockey in Brooklyn and wind up getting drum-rolled onto stages around the world, it has a certain appeal. For another thing, there was my promise to put myself in lights, onto videotape and into print to prove something to a woman who told me, in essence, that I was a dumb street kid with nice muscles. For another thing there was the matter of making a living, and all those trophies and a certain amount of fame were my most marketable asset. For still another and most important thing, I began to understand—and still understand, better than ever—that my main purpose in life is to promote health and fitness. You cannot do that by sitting quietly in a darkened corner.

So I launched my campaign on the unfamiliar turf of Detroit, Michigan, to become a successful entrepreneur, to become known, and to use my brain to do something with all those muscles.

One of the first things I learned is that you can't drive a Porsche 928 on the slushy streets of Detroit in the winter. So I found an old $500 rust-buster Cadillac. I put on my best suit and my best head and drove the rust-buster around town knocking on doors. Ninety-nine percent of them closed real quick. "That's great, Peter, you're a good-looking kid and you've got a lot of ambition and a lot of enthusiasm. But not today. Show me a track record."

It became a steady refrain. But I did my PT, I did my personal appearances for the fruit juice company, I scuffled and knocked on doors and I hung in there. Then one night my sister called and told me that Dad was dead. He had died, at peace, in the old apartment on Sixty-Seventh Street. Emphysema had left him too weak to fight back against a variety of illnesses. Pete Nielsen, the old New York Bell lineman, the macho father who took his son fishing and hunting, but who became enthusiastic mentor and mascot for a teenager who traipsed around the East Coast collecting trophies in a bikini, was gone.

I was so very sad and so very angry.

I loved this man who had once given me a simple little plaque with our family name on it, saying it was all he had to pass on to me, and that he knew I wouldn't dishonor it. He was full of life, yet he had helped to sap it from himself with what he put in his lungs and in his stomach. How could I think such a thing? How could I *not* think such a thing? How could he have done this to my sister, to my Mom, to me? How could I be blaming him for dying?

The plane wouldn't take me to New York until morning. In the middle of the night I went to the gym and had the most strenuous, awkward, bizarre workout of my life, and the only tearful one. I attacked the weights with the same fervor I attacked the karate classes Dad had dragged me to. In my head I was dedicating a workout to

Pete Nielsen. You don't dedicate a *workout* to somebody. But I did.
I guess if I were a painter, I would have done a canvas for him.

We buried Dad on Long Island. I told my Mom and sister that
I was the head of the household now, that in times of financial need
I would be there. And I flew back to Detroit with yet another pressing
motive for making something out of not much.

Except that Dad's death had changed the financial picture a bit.
There was life insurance, and Mom saw to it that part of it came to
me. I was determined to roll it over in a successful enterprise, to show
my family—and several other people—how Peter Nielsen could use
his brains as well as his biceps. There was enough money that I could
show some earnestness to investors, and could carry off my plan.

My plan was simple: to combine my training talents with the
medical community, to open a sports medicine/physical therapy facility
where the doctors could practice and I could help people my way.
Instead of sending money down the rat-hole like I did with my International Universe profits, I would put together something that would
be worthwhile, lasting and lucrative. I anted up about $6,000 for
blueprints, and a few thousand for other preparations. I found three
backers and committed $150,000 to landlords, construction people,
equipment vendors—and signed more documents than I had ever seen
in my life. I was about to enter the entrepreneurial world with the same
enthusiasm, but at considerably more depth, than the day I dropped
in at Studio 54. The day before Thanksgiving I was getting ready to
fly back to Brooklyn for a celebration when one of my backers called.

"Peter, you know that $20,000 check I gave you?"

"Yeah."

"Well, it's gonna bounce."

Backers back out of deals all the time. Learning that fact, however, was not exactly a big consolation. Thanksgiving in Brooklyn was
a day for heavy thought, and about as close as I've ever come to giving
up all the dreams. Instead, I went back to Detroit for a meeting with
a friend who was going to try to put another partnership together.

This is where I met Charlie Baughman, a guy who became
virtually my second father and who turned my world around. You
will have noticed by now that several people have turned my world
around—from Dr. Imperato to Julie Levine right on to Charlie

Baughman. I don't believe that to be an accident. Some people are graced by more good fortune than others, and I have had more than my share. But I believe that *much* good fortune comes from putting your eye on the prize and going for it. We can also use images about choosing the easy path or the difficult path, or a thousand bromides about hard work. The point is, nobody but a burglar or a salesman is going to find you sitting on your couch. If you're out there scouting, you'll find opportunity. Even then, too many people sidestep it instead of meeting it head-on.

Anyway, my persistence led me to Charlie Baughman, an ex-Ford Motor executive running his own company who—more than anybody—led me into the business world.

"What a day, kid," he said at that first meeting, "I've got to solve all these problems. Wait until you get older. You don't know how lucky you are right now."

"You only think you have problems, Mr. Baughman," I said, "I have to raise $75,000 in 10 days or my business plan is going down the tubes and I'm gonna be $150,000 in debt."

I didn't say it as a whine. I was just leaving the office where we met, and I almost said it kiddingly, to commiserate with him on his own bad day. Charlie motioned me back and said, "Tell me about it."

So Charlie learned the whole sad story of the backers who took a hike from my plans for a clinic. He asked me to lunch the next day and we talked for two hours. And then he told me that I was wet behind the ears, that I was a diamond in the rough, and that I had just met a lot of the wrong people. Except that I had met some of the right people, like the accountant who was carrying me on the books even though I couldn't pay the bill—and was therefore able to supply the detailed prospectus that Charlie wanted to see.

He was impressed. "You've got the makings of a pretty good team, kid," Charlie said. "I'm going to see if I can get you a loan."

There was another lunch, this time with two bankers. Charlie told me to wear a suit, and I was sweating into it profusely as the questions flowed over the appetizers. Then Charlie said, "Before we eat, why don't we let Peter relax a little." One of the bankers put an envelope on a dish in front of me. It contained a check, made out to me, for $75,000.

"All you have to do is sign this," the banker said. "Mr. Baughman signed the rest of the papers. He guaranteed the note."

I'm not naive enough to suggest that hard work and commitment are going to put $75,000 on a plate in front of you tomorrow. But I want to tell you that there are some very nice people out there. And that if you walk what you talk, if you get up off the couch and persist, you're liable to meet some of them. Charlie became not only a business partner but a mentor who taught me more business savvy in six months than I had learned in my life to date. Between my penchant for turning adversity into a positive, and Charlie's financial and educational backing, we put together a first-class team: me, Charlie, my accountant, and my lawyer.

The clinic happened. It almost doesn't matter that after three years I was out of it, at a loss, in what amounted to a hostile takeover by the MDs. I already had opened the first Eye of the Tiger—despite my own fears of overextending—because Charlie said, "Hey, all these people that get better at the clinic are going to need a place to work out, right?" That first fitness center turned out to be a major success. I recently sold it, and—following my own ideas of how a good gym should be equipped and operated—more Peter Nielsen Eye of the Tiger fitness centers are on the franchise horizon. I still train, and train others, at the original gym in suburban Detroit. Well, not quite the original; that was my grandmother's basement, where there definitely wasn't any tiger-striped carpet.

Other enterprises, all aimed at becoming an effective spokesman for fitness, began to sprout like mushrooms in the woods.

I told you that I eat, sleep and breathe fitness. I probably say "I walk what I talk" more often than I should, but that is very important to me. Especially since I talk a *lot:* feebies for the National Foundation for Ileitis and Colitis, which leads research into Crohn's; speeches to school groups about drugs and about fitness; motivational talks to business groups. Once I lectured to a skeptical meeting of MDs who were definitely not looking forward to an anecdotal message from an at-home graduate of Fort Hamilton High. But by the end of my speech, many were waiting to thank me for reminding them that—though they were the experts on medicine—the holistic approach is the path toward health. I never give quite the same speech twice, and I never use notes. I find out what makes each audience different, and I try to reach them the best way I know how. Everybody tells me it works.

Despite that macho promise I made standing beside an empty refrigerator, my picture has never appeared on a billboard, and I'm not aware of my name in lights blinding anybody. But I began to find my mug in a Detroit newspaper quite often as its health writer developed columns on fitness. I wrote a book for kids, called *Growing Up Strong*. WDIV-TV, the NBC affiliate in Detroit, hired me for a fitness segment on their morning newscast. It has been fun—and useful, I think, because seldom do I talk about weightlifting. I'm more likely to talk about getting the most out of lawn mowing or (this is Detroit, remember) shoveling snow.

A few years ago I launched the Peter Nielsen brand of vitamins and supplements, a quality product packaged to my specifications, but which wasn't going anywhere. Charlie said, "Let's put it on TV, with an 800 number." Next thing I know I'm on one of those cable infommercials and—zoooom—sales got serious.

Besides, I met Cindy at the ad agency that did the commercial. She became the fourth member of the team, the one who is with me day and night. No one would have been more amazed than chocolate-loving Cindy that first day at the ad agency if someone had told her that very shortly she would be into a new lifestyle, designing interiors and ads for Eye of the Tiger, broiling chicken twice a day, doing PT herself, and putting on a bikini to pose with me on the cover of a national muscle magazine. Motown has been good to me in a thousand ways, but none as great as Cindy.

It would be fair to say that the only blinding lights anybody has to be concerned about are the ones shining in my own eyes. I have a big-time company pursuing endorsement and licensing deals for me. We're talking deals for a series of exercise videos. They tell me I have a world of opportunity in the motivational speaking arena. I'm the first guy I know from Sixty-Seventh street to publish a book. Not to worry about the blinding lights, though. I've learned that sometimes things happen and sometimes they don't, and the most important things have nothing to do with bright lights. I've become, in the words of one pastor who made an impression on me, "evenly yoked." Family, career, self-worth, the worth of others—all represent a slice of my outlook, and I try to give them all my full attention. Fitness and health are the harness that reaches from everybody's yoke to the load they're pulling, and that's where I want to make an impact.

In much of the rest of this book we'll be talking about the nuts and bolts of fitness. But it's vital that you not overlook the grand design, the master blueprint. That has nothing to do with how to perform certain exercises, or how many grams of fat are in your lunch. It has to do with attitude, with an understanding that the body you live in is temporary housing, that it's yours for maybe seven decades if you're fortunate, and that the quality of life for you and those you love will largely be determined by how much you invest in upkeep. The beauty part is that it doesn't cost a cent of cash.

That's why I've taken up all this space telling you my own story. I want you to learn something not just about physical fitness, but about yourself. By telling my own story, I'm putting a mirror in front of you so you can see not Peter Nielsen, but yourself—and maybe some other people you love. I don't want you to see a bodybuilder's musculature in the mirror, I just want you to see a reflection of the best you can be. I want you to see someone who is getting the most out of life, someone whose day is a series of events met with energy rather than fatigue, someone for whom *all* time is quality time.

How does the story of a Brooklyn kid with a strange disease who wound up flexing his muscles under a spotlight relate to *every* reader, as I'm convinced it does?

Most importantly, I've learned one big lesson. Life is a place where we all make mistakes. Even if we make fewer than our share of mistakes, fate will toss some obstacles in our way. The greatest thing about life is that if the mistake isn't too costly, we can keep trying until we get it right. If the obstacle isn't too big, we can keep trying until we get past it. The mistakes that millions of Americans make with their bodies are far too costly to correct years down the road. You cannot daily poor junk into your stomach, alcohol into your veins, smoke into your lungs and your butt onto the couch—and then expect to make a minor course correction somewhere down the line.

My life, and this book, are dedicated to helping you stop making mistakes so costly that they'll kill you, and to putting you on a *lifetime* course correction.

You don't need—nobody *needs*—a body that is as fine-tuned as mine. It's what I do for a living. But all the things I do to the max— nutritionally, in terms of exercise, in terms of mental outlook—can be adapted to a healthy lifestyle even if your primary focus is selling stocks or hanging drywall or arguing cases before juries or raising a family. Whatever your focus, fitness will sharpen the picture.

In a minute, we'll get on to the nuts and bolts. First, I want to tell you about the Eye of the Tiger.

8

About That Song

Tell me a kid from Bensonhurst wasn't going to relate to those early
Rocky films. No way. If nothing else, Philadelphians—or at least Sly
Stallone—even sound like they're from Brooklyn.

It wasn't the films that really got to me, though. It was a song,
the one from *Rocky II*. I first heard it before the movie came out in
1979, when I was working out at Julie's and first started getting into
competition. The song got to me in a big way.

I wore beat-up sneakers and I ran on asphalt that had potholes
a person could disappear in. The holes in my sneakers I dealt with
by putting on extra pairs of socks. But it wasn't the blue-collar champion theme that I related to so strongly; it had to do with Crohn's,
this obstacle I was trying to turn into a positive. I had *The Eye of the
Tiger*, just like the song said. I was competitive for life; the big prize
for me was just being healthy. Except that the song came out just
when I had my first serious relapse, and I latched onto that song
almost immediately. It kept growing on me, and became my life's
theme.

I remember being sick, and being back at the family apartment—the nest I often returned to when things weren't right. I
remember being upstairs, and a friend coming over to visit, and I
remember getting cramps so bad I thought I'd need an ambulance.
Mom wanted me to go to the corner store to get something for dinner,

and there I sat with the onset of panic and denial descending on me all over again.

How could this be happening? I had already won a major teen-age bodybuilding championship. I thought I had my health back. I had been feeling great. And no I was terrified that I couldn't hold me bowels long enough to get to the corner and back. Was I so fragile that even after all that work I could just suddenly, without warning, fall apart?

The bottom line was that I had been taking my health for granted again, not really watching what I ate, thinking—with an IQ of about 50—that if a body looks great on the outside everything must be great on the inside. I was breaking up with a girlfriend, a car I liked a lot had just been stolen—and now I was having a relapse. Perception and reality can be such different animals.

And then I heard this song about how quickly we can change, how easy it is to trade passion for glory. Much of my still-young life has been devoted to learning that lesson. I like to think that by now I've learned it fairly well.

Crohn's was a great reminder. I had three major setbacks in 10 years. Each time, I thought I had arrived, that the disease was in permanent remission, and each time nature reminded me that life is short and the path is tricky. Corny as it may sound, that song from *Rocky II* meant a lot to me each time I found myself back again at square one and bleeding.

The worst time of all was 13 days before I got on a plane to Belize to win the title that got me all that hardware and, indirectly, all that cash. It was—BOOM—like somebody chopped off my kneecaps. This time I was heavy into training, eating exactly the right foods—and still here comes the Crohn's. Unbelievable. I remember looking at myself in the mirror, slapping myself in the face and saying: "There's no way you can get sick." Guess again. I calmed down, but I was not in the best of health when I won that trophy.

This is why I talk about mistakes *and* obstacles. You can remove mistakes from your life. You can fight obstacles, but you can't prevent them. I'm not guaranteeing anyone that if you take care of yourself and develop the most positive mental outlook that you won't be hit by a debilitating disease. Only God knows that. You could get hit by a bus tomorrow. I had read the recipe and I was following instructions, and still I got hit again. That's the kind of obstacle that makes you start feeling sorry for yourself, and that's why I like that song so much.

It says everything you need to hear: I went the distance and I'm not going to quit; I'm back on the street and I'm here to win, and I'm going to bring it home for all the right reasons.

That's the Eye of the Tiger that I see at bodybuilding championships, where you can pick out the winners in their gazes better than in their muscles. I see it in successful people in all kinds of endeavors. Call it discipline or motivation or whatever you want. I'm sure the heavy thinkers have better words for it. "Eye of the Tiger" is good enough for me.

I've got it because I was blessed with adversity, and because I followed through on it. Being sick gave me tremendous desire to be well. It motivated me to learn how the body works, how to use it, and what to put in it. I work out. I eat well. I have confidence, and because I look good I have even more confidence. It's a total package: priorities, values, self-love, love for others, health, fitness—all of a sudden you're running on all cylinders. You're in *overdrive*.

My most important message is this: There are many components to that total package, but *nobody* can have the Eye of the Tiger unless fitness is part of the package. *Anybody* can have the Eye of the Tiger if they start by doing the best they can for the frame they're going to have to live in 24 hours a day, cradle to grave.

Part Two

Nutrition: Where It All Begins

9

Going Against the Flow

The neighborhood *a la carte* pork store in Bensonhurst is a perfect symbol for the disaster area otherwise known as America's eating habits. No offense to my friend Louis, whose family runs a *fine* pork store, but just one look at the crowd lined up along the sidewalk on a Friday afternoon is enough to choke your arteries and, meanwhile, send you off to the Big and Tall shop to buy new clothes.

Delicacy lies in the eye of the beholder. Here are some of the delicacies for which the good citizens of Brooklyn *take a number*, get in line, and jostle their way forward to animal-fat heaven: Prosciutto, spicy ham marbled with golf-ball-sized circles of fat. Sausages, in dozens of sizes and flavors, all guaranteed to heat up dripping with fat. Brajole, a concoction consisting of fat wrapped in fat—a jelly roll of pork and mozzarella. Amazing. The mind, and the taste buds, can be trained to favor almost any kind of food. Even when large, sustained doses of it will slow you down, balloon your bodyfat, and maybe kill you.

They call America the Melting Pot. Nutritionally speaking, it's more like the Rendering Pot. Everything boils down to fat. We take the *worst* nutrition of our various cultures and share it with one another, in profusion. Not just the Italians, but all the sausage-making cultures offer up their bratwurst and other cholesterol-stuffed tubes. African-Americans taught us how to yearn for our chicken to be fried.

73

The French taught us how to take a perfectly nutritious meal and drown it in dairy fat. The Mexicans taught us how to find vegetable protein in a mixture of corn and beans; but then they wrecked the recipe by refrying the beans in lard. Together, we savor every greasy variation—right down to the cross-cultural common denominator: the burger with fries.

We are the richest country in the world. But we have the poorest eating habits.

We invented high technology and public education. But we eat like illiterates.

We have the money and the time to be the healthiest people in the world. But we are perhaps the least fit of all nations.

We face a health-care crisis, with medical bills eating up a disastrous and growing portion of our wealth. We spend billions of dollars trying to repair bodies destroyed by junk food, fast food, fatty food, alcohol, cigarettes and lack of exercise—and still can't begin to fix the damage. We never will, really, no matter how many more billions we spend on coronary bypasses and cancer surgeries. The incredible irony is that we could slash this suffocating repair bill by spending *less* money on junk to put in our stomachs. Only a dunce would be surprised at the repair bill for a 100,000-mile car that has never been maintained. Where's the surprise if the mechanic, after using up $500 of your paycheck, still can't get your junker running right?

That's just looking at it in terms of dollars and cents. How we *feel*, how much quality we get out of each day can't be measured on the bottom line. Or can it? Somebody probably has done a study suggesting that trillions of dollars in productivity gets lost to poor nutrition and other unhealthy habits that leave us rundown, unalert, uninterested.

Who's to blame? Every out-of-shape individual, of course, whether he or she is carrying around visible flab or it is hidden in clogged arteries. Nobody puts a gun to your head and forces you to spend $2 for a big bag containing two cents worth of potatoes and three cents worth of oil. Nobody forces those chips down your throat while you sit and watch TV. Well, at least not exactly. Powerful forces do aid and abet this nutritional felony, and it doesn't hurt to be aware of them. It's necessary, in fact, to be conscious of all the baloney that gets shoved at you day and night in modern America. Otherwise, you'll eat it.

First of all, there is that cultural influence, our various heritages of fatty food. Of course, every culture has its share of healthy foods, too. But remember, we're affluent; so we pour grease on the perfectly healthy pasta. Americans can afford it, so they choose the "reward" foods—the ones we're supposed to have only on rare occasion—almost every time they eat. From my own heritage, I can assure you that alfredo sauce was not something the peasants ladled on their pasta every night. Even pizza picked up 95 percent of its fat calories only after it was Americanized.

Second of all, as the 21st Century approaches, chances are excellent that you were raised by parents who were not exactly nutritional role models. Nutrition is a modern, evolving science. Only a few decades ago, researchers were missing important pieces of the puzzle (a few are still missing). The world of processed, packaged, sodium-laden, nutrient-robbed, greasy food was a done deal before nutritional knowledge caught up with it. Some families are into a second generation that has no idea what it means to eat fresh produce—or even to sit down together for a home-cooked meal.

Third of all, we're into the fifth decade of commercial television. Fred Flintstone selling cocoa-choco-whatevers to wide-eyed five-year-olds who are developing permanent lifetime eating habits. Basketball stars who—as the commercials make perfectly clear—developed their ability to jump into the sky by drinking soda pop. Role models of every stripe selling their souls for the almighty buck. They're really selling the souls of those kids, whose present and future health is endangered by the commercials. Is that a far-out, left-field viewpoint? I don't think so. The commercial messages must work, or the junk-food conglomerates wouldn't spend millions to produce them.

Fourth of all, the educational system—meaning the schools, the household environment, the media—has not done its part to erase nutritional ignorance. You don't have to go far to find someone who thinks a soupbowl of ice cream is a healthy thing because it's made with milk—"nature's most perfect food." We still have millions of people walking around who think that a monstrous chunk of meat in one two-ton meal is the way to "get your protein." We are a nation that eats most of its food out of packaging that misleads, or tells outright lies. Most of us don't know how to read the fine print—and even the fine print doesn't tell the whole story.

That sounds pretty grim. But the answers to a couple of obvious questions about nutrition should paint a brighter picture for you, if you're truly interested in cleaning up your act.

So who do you trust?

You trust yourself. You learn how to make intelligent choices, and you put yourself in charge. That's a good feeling—avoiding manipulation, being free of all the baloney and using your brain to make sound, healthy decisions about your own body.

Does that mean you have to drive out into the country in search of organically gown vegetables, and live on steamed cauliflower seven times a week?

Of course not. One of the benchmarks of a healthy diet is its *variety*. It *is* trickier than shouting "Two cheeseburgers!" into a drive-in speaker. You can't eat today's typical American diet and be fit; but you don't have to eat sawdust, either.

Can I eat myself fit; or do I have to exercise?

Nobody can be fit without regular exercise. Obviously. But it's no accident that the exercise section of this book falls between the nutritional and mental discipline sections. The physical work of building muscles and/or cardiovascular endurance is just one part of the package. All three elements are necessary. All three rely on each other. So I hate to single out any one of the three. If I had to, it would be *nutrition*. If someone is dumb enough to condemn himself or herself to the life of a couch potato—or if disability leaves them no choice—good nutrition will still improve health and fitness. And, to get back to the question, *good nutrition will lead you toward exercise more than exercise will lead you toward good nutrition.*

That is a humongously important fact. Good nutrition is going to make you *look good* faster than exercise is going to make you look good. Not only will you decrease your bodyfat nutritionally, but you will need less sleep, your insulin level will be stabilized and your metabolism won't take you yo-yo-ing and roller-coastering through the day. Your body will feel better-tuned, and you'll have more energy for whatever you want to do—including exercise. Good nutrition alone is not enough, but it is a tremendous positive factor for fitness.

Mental discipline is something I'd like to say a few words about separately at the end of the book. But it's impossible to entirely separate mental discipline from nutrition. You cannot pick up new eating habits the way you would pick up a suit from the cleaners. We are talking about a change of life. We are talking about a new personal understanding of reality, based on what food does to and for your body—not based on TV commercials, or on the status involved in paying big bucks for lobster Newburg and New York-style cheese-cake at your favorite restaurant. Nutrition takes an old truism—"You get what you pay for"—and stands it on its head. The fact is, you buy good nutrition with your brain and with your mental discipline, not with your wallet. You can eat well for pennies, if you choose.

One restaurant I know in New York serves a well-marbled steak the size of a dump truck. The beef practically hangs over the table. It costs a *lot* of money. If the guy in the $1,000 suit with the steak knife in his hand is a good planner, he has drawn up a will. Because his idea of good nutrition is going to see to it that his heirs are spending the old man's money a lot sooner than he ever intended. Somebody at the next table, or at a little place down the street where the tab will be a whole lot smaller, is eating a tasty but healthy meal and enjoying it every bit as much. Why? Because they invested enough mental discipline to go against the flow and develop a new palate, one that's based on nutritional reality.

Go against the flow is worth repeating. Because, in a nation with lousy eating habits, that is exactly what you must do. Going against the flow is never easy. Just look at the progress that has been made in cutting back on smoking. Now that it's cool not to smoke, there are converts all over the place. You can go *with* the flow and quit. As if we haven't known for years and years what a stupid and destructive habit tobacco is. When serious numbers of people look at a cheese-burger and an order of chili fries with the same disgust that they look at a cloud of cigarette smoke, then it'll be a whole lot easier to break the junk food habit.

In the '90s, it's hard to imagine anybody being *totally* ignorant of the good-nutrition message. Most everybody talks the language, sort of. Fewer people are buying steaks the size of dump trucks. But mostly the message gets garbled into concoctions like diet pop and light beer, soyburgers topped with cheese, and grocery shelves full of packaged products with "25 percent less fat and sodium!!!" (still leaving you with 200 percent too much of both). The sad truth is that most of us remain functionally illiterate when it comes to nutrition. What do I mean? I mean the woman I saw in a Wendy's trying to do the right thing. She pretty much symbolizes where we are in terms of what we put in our stomachs.

For starters, she was in a fast-food joint. That's no particular rap on Wendy's. They all present a challenge to anyone who wants to eat right. And did she ever try. She ordered the grilled chicken breast sandwich. Great choice. Lots of protein, minimal fat. She ordered a whole wheat bun. Great choice. Tons more nutrition than the empty white stuff. She even ordered a baked potato, getting her complex carbohydrates without the deep-fat coating of french fries. She was on her way to her table as a winner! But then she made a fatal stop at the condiment counter. What did she do? She poured ranch dressing all over her chicken and all over her potato. Instant disaster. More calories, and more fat, than her chicken and bun and potato put together.

Of course, she could have chucked the whole thing and gotten a salad with "light" Italian dressing. But then she would be consuming 1,200 milligrams of sodium, and the cottonseed oil in the recipe—while representing a low level of fat—would produce cholesterol in her body, helping to clog her arteries.

It's a mine field out there, all right. With no quick fixes, and no substitute for knowledge. A lot of nutrition consultants and weight-loss entrepreneurs would like to make it sound easy, almost like good nutrition is some kind of temporary inconvenience. Anyone who sells you that idea is selling you a crock.

Weight loss—meaning loss of bodyfat—is just one aspect of good nutrition. But it's a paramount concern for millions of Americans who spend billions of dollars in futile attempts to get weight off and keep it off. Chances are that bodyfat loss is one of your own concerns, one of the reasons you're reading this book. Chances are that you have tried not just one "diet," but many. Well, let me say up front that the word "diet"—as most people understand it—ought to be banned from the language. *No* temporary nutritional regimen can get you in shape, let alone keep you in shape.

Here is basically what I tell potential clients who come to me and ask me about nutritional counseling and personal training:

"It has taken you maybe 30 years to get the way you now look and feel. It will take a lot more than 30 days to turn it around. I'm not a magician. I'm not God. I can pass on to you the education and experience I've acquired. There's only one right way. I can give you the nuts and bolts. I can tell you how to do it. But until you get into the program mentally and emotionally, you are not going to see one physical change.

"After I talk with you and give you my written analysis, and take your $150, that analysis won't be worth the paper it's written on if *you* don't implement it. That piece of paper gives you no sympathy, no empathy. I've made my fee honestly, and I'd like to see you lose weight; but only 30 percent of the people I've counseled follow through and do it. The successful ones get into the mental discipline part of it. And they lose weight big-time.

"You can't have people going from 300 pounds to 180, going from emotionally distressed to Mr. Brooklyn, making these kinds of changes unless you're preaching the right message. I am. But the bottom line is that the successful ones had the *desire* to do it. You need to make a commitment not with me, but with *yourself.*"

That's the unvarnished truth.

I do want to help you find the will to make a lifestyle change. Nutritionally speaking, like the wise cliche says, I want to help you eat to live instead of living to eat. I want to provide some of the inspiration to get you into your own personal fitness program, in whatever way works best for you. But you know what they say about 10 percent inspiration and 90 percent perspiration. You have to do your own perspiring. You have to eat your own meals. You have to develop your own Eye of the Tiger.

That's one reason I used Part One to tell my story. Parts of it were not fun to tell. I like to think that a lot of readers will be smart enough if not inspired enough to say: "Hey, this guy's no genius. He had a debilitating disease. Damned near killed him. So he learned the hard way, by necessity. I think I'll get in tune with my body now, before it's too late."

If you are really ready to make that decision, you'll find that I'm about to give you the most basic, sane, realistic nutritional advice I know. No gourmet recipes, no emotional babysitting. Just the nuts and bolts. Because when you get a better grasp of *why* you should follow a healthy regimen, you're liable to be better motivated to get with it.

I learned all this stuff the hard way, for hard reasons. If you're lucky, your only reasons for learning it are to live longer, live better and fully enjoy your short little run on this planet.

That ought to be motivation enough.

10

What's In It for Me?

When you look at a well-prepared dish of food, what you see is something delicious like shrimp scampi or linguini with clam sauce. Another way of looking at it would be to see complex carbohydrates and cholesterol. The difference between those two visions is huge. I don't want you to lose the pleasure that comes with the first vision, and there's no reason you should. But if you want to be nutritionally fit, you'll have to start seeing the world of food through both lenses.

Looking through the analytical lens, I know exactly what goes into my body every day. I know by the gram, and in some cases by the milligram, what nutrients are stoking my fire. I'm an extreme case at the moment, because I have a bodybuilding competition coming up. But even if I weren't preparing for an event, even if you could tell me today that in no way would my physical appearance ever again have any bearing on my career, I would remain more aware of what I eat than 99 percent of the population. That's because in the last 15 years I've learned from experience that the benefits reach far beyond developing a body that you can display on a stage.

I don't know how far you plan to go down the road toward personal nutrition awareness. Even if you're dead serious, you won't have to count grams of protein quite as closely as I do. You won't have to be as stopwatch-precise as I am with my meals. You won't have to pass up quite as many "reward" treats as I do. But whether you are into a serious athletic regimen or barely exercising, you should have at least a working knowledge of basic nutrients. You should know what they do for you and to you. You should know how to structure a healthy dietary regimen to fit your tastes and your lifestyle.

So let's use this chapter to have a basic look, through that second lens, at all the stuff—good and bad—that you put in your stomach.

WATER

H_2O is the "forgotten" nutrient. Many people are dehydrated and don't even know it. Not everyone who is tired, moody and fatigued is dehydrated, of course, but those are symptoms.

In one sense, water isn't a nutrient at all. Nutrients—the raw materials for fueling our bodies and building new cells—are found in food. But water is crucial to virtually every basic function of the body, from temperature regulation to blood circulation, metabolism, the immune system and waste elimination. The fact that something so basic can be so misunderstood, or ignored, shows just how far out of touch the average person is with his or her own body and its maintenance.

Take, for example, the matter of weight control—which always seems to be the one area where the average American picks up at least a passing interest in nutrition.

If you are overweight, or if you have fluid retention problems, you should be drinking *more* water. If you keep your body adequately supplied with water, it will actually speed up your metabolism. When the body is not being given enough water, it sees that as a threat to survival and—like a camel—begins to hang onto every drop. Drink more water, and the body will release the excess. Water also suppresses appetite, and naturally helps the body metabolize stored fat—so overweight people, with a larger metabolic load, need more water than thin people.

Every body, thin or fat, needs plenty of water every day. The average person loses about two cups daily through perspiration (temperature control), even without unusual physical exertion. Another two cups disappear in the respiratory process. The intestines and kidneys together use about six cups a day. That's about 10 cups total— not counting water loss through perspiration during any heavy exercise.

Some of that water loss is replaced through the food we eat, liquid or solid. The bottom line, however, is that the average person should be drinking at least six to eight cups of *water* each day. To be more specific, divide your bodyweight by two. That gives you the number of ounces of water you should be drinking. Divide that by eight to get the number of cups.

Be grateful to your kidneys, nature's filtering department. If you could somehow survive without them, you'd need to drink *2,500 gallons* of water every day just to flush out the system.

The fact is, millions of Americans don't come close to drinking their daily quota of water. Their rationale is that the oceans of pop, coffee, beer and liquor/soda combinations they knock down every day will do the trick. Well, there are some serious problems with that idea. Alcohol and caffeine, besides depleting the body of vitamins and minerals, are natural diuretics—meaning they actually lead to fluid elimination, and dehydration.

There are many degrees of dehydration, of course. We're not talking about someone dying in the desert as his body runs dry. Lesser levels of dehydration occur when you don't take in enough water to replace all that's lost through breathing, urination and exercise. You don't have to be perspiring profusely or urinating frequently to be losing water. If you work in a stuffy house or office building, you lose large amounts of liquid invisibly. You can lose two pounds of water in the rapidly circulating cabin air of a three- or four-hour airplane flight. Stress, as well as alcohol and caffeine, acts as a diuretic. In other words, you can be dehydrating yourself on a *normal* day.

Speaking athletically—or in terms of any kind of physical performance—seventy-five percent of muscle tissue is water. Dehydrate a muscle by three percent and you lose 10 percent of contractual strength and eight percent of speed. Dehydration increases blood volume. Thicker, more concentrated blood stresses the heart. Your arteries become less able to provide muscles with nutrients and oxygen, and to eliminate accumulated wastes. So you don't need to be a scientist, rocket or otherwise, to figure out that dehydration is a common cause of poor athletic performance.

On the more cerebral side, dehydration can produce a minuscule but crucial shrinkage of the brain. Deprive yourself of enough water and your concentration and coordination will be affected.

In other words, you need those six to eight cups a day whether you're pumping iron in a gym or crunching numbers at a desk.

People often tell me: "No problem; I drink tons of water with my meals." Well, that is *exactly the wrong way* to consume your quota of water. It dilutes your food and makes for less efficient absorption of nutrients. If you drink milk, that is OK with meals because milk becomes a semi-solid in the stomach. But you should avoid water beginning 15 minutes before a meal; and after a meal you should give your stomach 30 to 60 minutes to begin the digestive process.

Thirst, by the way, is a lousy barometer of whether or not you need water. Best to make water a habit. (You'll find that 90 percent of the battle with a dietary regimen is nothing but habit, so give it a chance.) Best of all, water is almost habit-*forming*. It isn't at all excessive to carry a squirt bottle with you, and to drink water throughout the day.

Once you become water-conscious, you'll become fascinated by the stuff. In virtually any building in the United States, you can turn a little handle and gallons of water come out—for pennies. Meanwhile, down at the supermarket, other kinds of water sell for several dollars a bottle. You need to know a little about both varieties.

Fluoride, for example, has been endorsed by the American Dental Association, and I haven't seen anything to convince me that fluoride in tap water will cause increased rates of disease. But, especially with children, I sometimes wonder if there isn't a fluoride overload in toothpaste, mouthwash and tap water. Chlorine, in sufficient dosage, is known to cause cancer. What's the bottom line with these chemicals in tap water? I wouldn't begin to judge whether you or I should avoid the water that comes out of any particular faucet. But I like to be aware of the fact that it's not a mountain stream pouring into my drinking glass.

Thousands of subdivisions and communities get their water from wells. Some wells produce hard water, some soft. In either case, it might have a peculiar taste. Chemically softened water is actually worse for drinking than straight tap water. Calcium and magnesium salts are replaced by sodium salts, adding as much as 100 milligrams of extra sodium per quart. Hard water, by contrast, contains relatively high amounts of distilled mineral salts that may help *prevent* heart disease.

In any case, even if your source of tap water is 100 percent pure and palatable, it might not be so pure by the time it gets to your kitchen faucet. Many Americans still are served by ancient underground pipes that add copper and lead to the water. A single gallon of gasoline, if allowed to seep into the water supply, could contaminate it for an entire small community.

What all this means is that home water purification is something worth looking into. A $15 filter system over your tap isn't a bad bet. If you're super serious about it, you could have a sample of your tap water tested. Or, more practically, you could do a little investigating to find out what kind of regular testing is done by your local officials. And maybe ask for a look at the results.

Bottled water is another story. Just because it costs a lot of money and portrays a pleasant rural scene on the label doesn't necessarily mean it's anything special. One survey showed that 93 brands of bottled water were being sold in New York. In most cases, the consumer couldn't really tell where the water came from or what was in it.

I always suggest that people launching a dietary regimen—a new eating lifestyle—start out drinking distilled water, at least for the first 90 days. Distilled water has many benefits, not the least of which being that it's relatively cheap. It helps flush out any unwanted mineral deposits from the body, especially if you've been drinking hard water for years. It is, literally, *pure* water; and it functions almost like a detox agent.

You could say that distilled water is "empty," but that's just fine. You ought to be getting your calcium and magnesium from green leafy vegetables anyway.

Drinking plenty of distilled water does exactly what those daily six to eight cups are supposed to do, no more and no less. It helps the body's organs go about their business. It's the lubricating oil of your personal engine. Your high-octane fuel—or low-octane junk—will come from the food that you eat.

FAT

We might as well put the big negative right at the head of the list. Eating *some* fat in your food is essential to your health. But mostly—overwhelmingly, in the case of the average American diet— fat is big-time bad news.

Scores of harmful and even fatal results have now been linked, solidly, to high-fat diets—cancer, hypertension, cardiovascular disease and poor absorption of calcium from the small intestine, to name a few. Those risks are real whether you are obese or your constitution and exercise load have kept your body in pretty good shape.

If weight loss is a concern, dietary fat is the Big Enchilada. The human body does a super job of converting excess dietary fat into excess bodyfat. Eating fatty foods is like mainlining pounds. In the case of fat, garbage in and garbage out would be a blessing. Instead, it's garbage in; period.

What this means is that most of what your grandparents told you may have been sound advice; but what they told you about carbohydrates was hogwash. "Starchy" foods do not put fat on your body. *Fat* (and sometimes even protein, as you'll see in a moment) puts fat on your body. Even refined carbohydrates, such as candy, are less "fattening" than fat.

Fat-wise, the simple step toward using that second, analytical lens to look at food is to remember that there is visible fat and there is invisible fat. If you look at an untrimmed T-bone steak, you can see the fat as clearly as the spare tire on a couch potato. In our mostly shallow nutrition-consciousness, we're eating a lot less T-bone steak these days. But there is invisible fat in almost every corner of the menu, and we're not doing a very good job of avoiding it.

Grandpa's advice on carbos may have been off-base, but apparently he didn't suffer for it. People who measure these things report that from 1910 to 1980, average per-capita daily fat consumption in the United States rose from 125 grams to 156 grams. Grandpa may have been a meat and potatoes man. But it's pretty clear that he was not a french fries man, a potato chips man, or a fast-food man. Today, when we should know better, the average American diet derives more than 40 percent of total calories from fat. You can find some loud debate on just how much fat we should be eating. But any way you slice the arguments, we're eating about *twice* as much fat as we should. You don't cut out that kind of fat surplus by eliminating one milk shake and one hamburger a week.

Fat is hidden in hundreds of foods, including most of America's most popular sandwiches and recipes. Margarine, butter, salad dressing, mayonnaise and fine oils account for 10 to 20 percent of the fat we eat. Red meat, poultry and fish account for 30 to 40 percent. Dairy products account for 15 to 25 percent. The rest comes from various sources such as nuts and eggs.

Almost everybody now is at least aware that there are three kinds of fat and two kinds of cholesterol, and that some are more user friendly than others. But most Americans don't retain much of that knowledge, and certainly don't act on it. They look only through that first lens, and they see the shrimp scampi instead of the fat and the cholesterol. The next few paragraphs include facts that *anybody* ought to know very well by now. Conversations I have every day with *health-conscious* clients convince me that isn't the case. So without going into great detail, we have to talk about what fat means nutritionally.

More than 90 percent of dietary fat arrives at the body in complex molecules consisting of three fatty acids: saturated, monounsaturated and polyunsaturated. Animal fats usually contain a high percentage of saturated fat. Keeping track of what kinds of fat you eat, however, is tricky. Beware, for example, snack foods whose labels proclaim "pure vegetable oil" as an ingredient. Coconut and palm oils contain even more saturated fatty acids than beef fat or lard. And don't be misled by "cholesterol-free" claims. Once digested, these oils do raise cholesterol levels in the blood. As you'll see, the simple—and effective—route is to limit your intake of fat of any kind. The fact is, that white stuff that borders your T-bone steak is fat; but so is the oil in your salad dressing.

Cholesterol is a wax-like substance that, in one form, clings to the walls of your arteries and makes them function like a water pipe gone bad. This can lead to heart attacks and strokes. Some studies suggest strongly that lowering levels of serum cholesterol also reduces the risk of cancer. Cholesterol is comprised of two groups of lipoprotein compounds—"high density" and "low density." HDLs have come to be known as the "good" cholesterol, because they actually draw the substance away from coronary arteries. LDLs are generally regarded as the predominant villain in heart disease. When your doctor tells you your cholesterol ratio, he is telling you what percentage of your cholesterol level is made up of HDLs. It's something worth checking.

A high intake of fat from red meats, eggs, dairy products and tropical oils—predominantly saturated—risks increased LDL (bad) cholesterol in the blood. It also increases the need for essential fatty acids, which can create a cycle leading to excessive bodyfat and other health problems.

Essential fatty acids are indeed essential, in small amounts. Without them, the body cannot properly process and use the fats you ingest. Polyunsaturated fats—found in grains, seeds, nuts, soy foods and some vegetables—provide sequences of fatty acids called the Omega 6's and the Omega 3's. Your body's cells use these fatty acids to form membranes and conduct nerve impulses. Fatty acids are involved in hormonal function, brain function, aerobic metabolism and sexual wellness. Infants and young children need to consume somewhat more fat than adults. So getting the proper fat in the proper amount is crucial. But with such a wide variety of foods on our tables, rarely does anyone need to worry about adding vegetable oils to his diet.

In truth, nutritional science is still uncovering the nuts and bolts of fat and how it works in our bodies. For example, we know that the molecules of unsaturated oils—when hydrogenated for use in cakes, cookies, chips and other snacks—are rearranged into an unnatural framework that may cause health problems, even though they remain unsaturated. Margarine is produced from polyunsaturated fat, and is a cholesterol-free substitute for butter. But its chemical makeup may cause it to be associated with other health problems. On the positive side, recent studies suggest that olive oil and flax oil can reduce high blood pressure, stimulate pancreas secretion and lower levels of the (bad) LDL without lowering the (good) HDL.

So what's the answer?

To remember that fat is fat. You want to avoid animal fat, of course. But generally you need to think in terms of reducing intake of all kinds of fat, and to consume approximately equal amounts of saturated, polyunsaturated and monounsaturated. A small but growing number of nutritional experts recommend that you limit fat intake to 10 to 15 percent of total calories. If you want to follow the more "reasonable" and prevalent guidelines and shoot for 20 to 25 percent of calories from fat, don't forget: Statistically that means you'll probably have to cut fat intake almost in half.

It's time to start reading labels, to buy a cookbook or two that lists fat content, and even to put a food scale on your kitchen counter. Self-education on the subject of nutrition, you'll find, will not only improve your health, but it will be intellectually rewarding. Believe it or not, it will also be fun.

And *you* will be in control.

CARBOHYDRATES

Carbos might be the most misunderstood nutrient. Complex carbohydrates are your body's best source of energy. And, contrary to several generations of folklore, complex carbohydrates should be the No. 1 item on the menu when you are trying to lose weight.

Complex carbohydrates—whole grain cereals, breads, oatmeal, brown rice, pasta, muffins, bagels, baked potatoes—usually are high in fiber. These "starches" provide the essential fuel—glucose, or blood sugar—for energy in every cell of your body. Glucose also helps maintain body temperature, regulate respiration, repair tissue and sustain the immune system.

Complex carbos are the high-octane fuel I keep talking about when I can't resist comparing the human body to a high-performance engine. Simple carbohydrates are the cheap gasoline from the generic pump. They give you a quick high and then fade, giving you insulin surges that make for a rough-running engine. The American Heart Association was among a group that recommended Americans cut back on refined carbohydrates—sugar and white flour—which have no real nutritional value, except that quick, phony high.

Complex carbos are digested more slowly and more efficiently. Just like the name suggests, burning up their calories is a more complex task for the digestive and metabolic systems.

Sugars and starches both are classified as carbohydrates because they have a chemical similarity. All carbohydrates, simple or complex, actually are made up of one or more simple sugars. The most prevalent are glucose, fructose and galactose. Any one of these three alone is a monosaccharide. Join two together and you have a disaccharide. Glucose plus fructose equals sucrose, or table sugar. Glucose plus galactose equals lactose—the milk sugar that my own body rebels against so violently.

Complex carbohydrates—starches—are in a way literally the sweetest of the bunch. That's because they are *poly*saccharides—a combination of more than two simple sugars. Some polysaccharides contain more than 1,000 glucose molecules linked together. Nature bundles up these simple sugars along with protein, fiber, vitamins, minerals and other nutrients to make a complex carbo. A plate of pasta or a baked potato is a whole lot more than "starch."

Consuming large amounts of simple sugars presents health and performance problems. Devoid of vitamins, minerals and fiber, they offer no nutritional fringe benefits whatever. Refined white sugar—sucrose—heads the list of empty calories. The simple molecules in sucrose require very little digestion and quickly take blood sugar levels above normal. Every office-working candy fiend knows the roller-coaster effect very well. It occurs when the pancreas secretes insulin to remove excess glucose from the blood, causing a *downswing* in blood sugar.

A high intake of refined sugars has been linked to elevated cholesterol levels, chromium deficiency, heart disease, diabetes and a laundry list of other problems. Alternatives such as fructose, maple syrup, honey or even juice concentrate are no bargain, either. Any energy from simple carbos that is not burned up immediately by your metabolism will be converted to fat. The simple fact is that excessive use of any sweetener is unhealthy.

The bad news about complex carbohydrates is that if you don't burn them up, they, too, will be converted to fat. The good news—and one of the most basic keys to planning what you put in your stomach—is that the energy from complex carbohydrates can be stored for *48 hours* before it is converted to fat. Is this an efficient energy source, or what? Think about it. It's like a little metabolic miracle. It's the reason that complex carbos are the energy key for a finely tuned athlete who is about to run a 100-mile ultramarathon, or for a couch potato who doesn't want his 6 p.m. pig-out to go straight to his waistline.

After the digestive system turns carbos into glucose, or blood sugar, any of this energy that goes to the muscle cells must be metabolized and stored as muscle glycogen. A muscle cell can store about 90 minutes' worth of glycogen. Simple arithmetic shows you the value of up to 48 hours' worth of stored energy from complex carbos. It's a little more complicated than that, of course, and we'll talk about it later when we get into exercise.

Just remember that complex carbohydrates are the master fuel, not the fat-forming taboo they once were thought to be.

PROTEIN

You might think that exercise builds muscle. Not exactly. Exercise actually *tears down* muscle tissue. Protein builds it back, bigger and stronger. You have to destroy muscle in order to build it. And you can't do that without protein.

Obviously, athletes and construction workers need more protein than office workers.

I just said a page or two ago that carbohydrates might be the most misunderstood nutrient. On the other hand, that honor might belong to protein. Generations of kids have had tons of red meat and peanut butter put down in front of them with the warning: "Here; you need your protein."

Yes, you do. But the odds are that you need less protein than you think. And it's 2-to-5 that you're eating your protein *at the wrong time*. Protein is the building block to muscle, but your body is very finicky about how much protein it will accept at once.

During digestion, protein is broken down into amino acids. Twenty-two amino acids are known to be vital, and nine are known to be essential—meaning the body cannot manufacture them from other amino acids. That means they must come from your diet. And, since protein cannot be stored in the body like complex carbohydrates, you need a new supply each day. Furthermore, you need protein *several times each day*.

Your body can utilize 35 to 40 grams of protein in a $2^{1}/_{2}$-hour period. That's about $1^{1}/_{2}$ chicken breasts. Any additional protein consumed within that $2^{1}/_{2}$-hour period *will be converted to fat*. Yes, you can get fat by eating protein. No matter how nutritious the meal is, no matter how well you trimmed a cut of beef or chicken, no matter that you broiled it instead of drowning it in fat. Protein is a wonderful, necessary nutrient; but you must ration it to your body or you'll just be adding blubber.

Besides that, any excess protein that your body does not convert to glucose for storage must be eliminated as toxic waste. Athletically, this reduces performance and endurance. Athlete or not, protein overdose will make you tired, increase blood acidity, dehydrate you and cause mineral loss—especially calcium. Meanwhile, excess protein consumption places a burden on your liver and kidneys.

In case you're wondering, yes, all those old training tables where an athlete "gets his protein" by chomping into one of those Godzilla-sized steaks are strictly from the Stone Age. After 30–40 grams, he is getting *zero* protein and consuming 100 percent fat or waste.

The protein secret for an athlete, or anyone who does strenuous exercise or labor, is to forget the whole idea of three square meals a day. You have to give your body protein in doses that it can handle. In my case, in training for a competition, I eat *six* carefully planned meals a day. I'll explain all that later in detail. You needn't be that stringent or that precise unless you're into bodybuilding or high-performance athletics. The basic principle applies to everyone, however: eating too much protein at once is worse than useless to your body.

There are many sources of protein. Red meat, in fact, supplies plenty of protein. But like most traditional sources of protein in the American diet, red meat also supplies too much fat. The same goes for all that peanut butter that mom encouraged you to eat, and to the yolks of all those eggs Americans chow down every morning. (Egg whites are another story; I eat them by the dozen.) Chicken breast is a good low-fat alternative. So is fish.

The body doesn't discriminate against vegetable protein, but putting a meal together is a lot trickier. Individual grains, legumes and vegetables lack adequate amounts of one or more essential amino acids. So the protein they supply is called "incomplete" protein. Vegetarians long ago learned to combine two or more foods to make a "complementary" protein, one that the body can utilize just as well as a steak or an egg—but without the fat. Beans and corn, for example, combine to make a complementary protein. Many Oriental dishes combine vegetables with a tiny (by American standards) amount of beef, poultry or fish. It's no longer a secret that Oriental populations suffer an enormously lower rate of the diseases associated with our fatty diet.

As you launch a healthy new nutritional regimen, one of your first steps will be to round up a few cookbooks that will show you hundreds of tasty ways to put together complementary proteins. You'll find that the basic recipe is to combine legumes (soybeans, lentils, kidney beans, blackeyed peas, chick peas, navy beans, pinto beans, split peas, lima beans and others) with grains such as barley, corn, buckwheat, rice, oats or wheat. It's delicious. It's inexpensive. And your fat consumption will head straight south.

Nutritional science has confirmed what some entire cultures have known for thousands of years: that the need for huge amounts of protein is a myth. I'll show you later how to calculate exactly the amount of protein you need to add to your diet as your physical activity rises. Athletes—and anyone who is building muscle by tearing it down—do need more protein.

VITAMINS (AND MINERALS)

You should know two things from the get-go: (1) I've had my own vitamin company for eight years; (2) I'm not writing this to sell you my vitamins. Vitamins obviously are something special to me, but so is this book. So let me say up front that Peter Nielsen is not the only person in the world with an ethical, well-planned line of vitamin supplements for sale.

The fact is, in a perfect world it would seldom be necessary to buy vitamin supplements—unless your doctor discovered a hereditary or illness-related deficiency. If you had lots of time to shop for produce and to prepare all your meals, or if you had a live-in cook, you could be reasonably assured that your diet would touch all the vitamin bases. The realities of modern lifestyles don't allow many people to fit that description.

Today, the overwhelming majority of the food consumed in America is at least treated with preservatives for shelf life. Worse yet, much of our food is processed and packaged. We live in a fast-food frenzy, with nutrients cooked out of our food. We consume huge quantities of fat and sugar calories that are empty to begin with. In that environment, you would be insane not to educate yourself about vitamins. A good place to start is with the myths and misconceptions, which are huge.

Vitamins are not wonder drugs. They are not food; you can't live on vitamins alone. That may sound like a dumb and unnecessary statement, but you might be surprised at the level of misunderstanding. Many people, for example, do think they can replace at least part of their food with vitamins. The fact is, the body cannot even assimilate vitamins without food. Pumping vitamin supplements into an empty stomach is the nutritional—and financial—equivalent of dumping them down the garbage disposal.

Vitamins contain no caloric value, no energy. They are no substitute for carbohydrates or protein or fat or water, or even for each other. You cannot become Mr. USA, or obtain the body of a fashion model, by skipping meals and popping vitamins. Not only do they supply no energy, but they are not a component of body structure.

Vitamins are not pep pills. They are substances that make the body operate in its peak *normal* fashion, not to hype it up and bring out unnatural performance. Just like protein, too much can be a bad thing—a very bad thing. An oversupply of B1, for example, can affect the thyroid gland and insulin production. Excess D can create an excess of calcium in the bloodstream. Megadoses of vitamin C wash out B12.

Simply put, vitamins are organic substances necessary for growth, vitality and general well-being. Vitamins regulate metabolism through the enzyme system. They are crucial to your chemical balance, and a single deficiency can impair your entire body. Anybody who has been eating sugar, white flour, canned or preserved food, restaurant food that has been reheated, or fast food that has been sitting under a heat lamp has *some* level of deficiency. Most refined breads and cereals are high in nothing but carbohydrates. Enriched? Enriched with what? White flour is produced by removing 22 natural ingredients and, generally, replacing them with three B vitamins, vitamin D, calcium and iron salts. What comes back at you is hardly the staff of life.

Your lifestyle, and even your address, can rob your body of some of the vitamins and minerals (more on them in a minute) that you do get from your diet. Smoking cigarettes depletes vitamin C. Synthetic vitamin D in milk can deplete magnesium. Smog cover in a city leaves its residents with less vitamin D than rural dwellers get from the sun. Alcohol depletes B vitamins. Oral contraceptives can decrease the body's ability to make use of several vitamins. If you are eating a high-protein diet, you need more B6. That's just a sample.

Obviously, the idea of taking vitamin supplements isn't something to reject out of hand. Vitamins are one of the six important nutrients (along with water, carbohydrates, protein, fats and minerals). A simple working definition of all six is: "absorbable components of food necessary for good health." Vitamins and minerals, because of their unique (some would say mysterious) role in that absorption, are a good place to get in a few words about the process. A quick refresher course on digestion will help you get that second lens in focus.

Digestion is a chemical process more intricate than the most high-tech widget you ever heard of. It's about food, but it's not about award-winning cuisine. It's about nutrients. Your body begins chemically processing your food the moment you put it into your mouth, where an enzyme in the saliva called ptyalin begins to split starches into simple sugars. It's a 12- to 14-hour process for food to move through the stomach and intestines.

Virtually all absorption of nutrients occurs in the small intestine. That much you remember from junior-high biology. What you may not remember, and may not have cared much about until now as an adult who wants to better understand his or her own nutrition, is the role played by a few other amazing organs.

The liver is a four-pound chemical factory. Once you're aware of its role and complexity, you'll think twice about punishing it with large doses of alcohol. The liver can modify almost any chemical structure sent its way, and it is a powerful detoxifying machine. It's also a blood reservoir and a storehouse for certain vitamins, digested carbohydrates and insulin, which is released to regulate blood sugar. Your liver manufactures your enzymes, your cholesterols and your vitamin A from beta-carotene. It plays a key role in digesting protein. And it produces bile, which contains salts that start the digestion of fats.

The gall bladder holds bile, modifies its chemicals and concentrates it tenfold. Just the sight of food can be enough to empty the gall bladder.

The pancreas provides your body's most important enzyme: insulin, which is injected into the bloodstream where it accelerates the burning of glucose. The pancreas also secretes enzymes into the digestive tract to help break down fats, starches and protein.

You start to get the picture of how complex and wondrous this whole body engine is. I'm not trying to write a biology text here, but it's important to get some of these biological basics into your mind—and *keep* them there. Start thinking of food as the fuel for this engine, and you'll be less susceptible to food impulses, to forgetting about looking through that second lens when you're contemplating beef Wellington or a cream puff or an evening of martinis.

Vitamins are an intricate part of the enzyme system I just described. So are minerals, another minuscule piece of our nutrient intake but without which vitamins cannot function or be absorbed. The body can synthesize a few vitamins, but it cannot synthesize any minerals—the most important of which are calcium, iodine, iron, magnesium, zinc and phosphorous. About 18 minerals are known to be required for body function and maintenance, but many of them remain a mystery. Recommended daily allowances have been established for only six of them.

So where do vitamin supplements come from, and why are they sold in so many forms?

Most vitamins are extracted from natural sources. Vitamin A, for example, is taken from fish liver oil. B complex comes from yeast or liver. Vitamin E is usually extracted from soybeans, wheat germ or corn.

Tablets are the most common because they are easier to store, and have a longer shelf life than powders or liquids. Capsules usually are used for supplementing oil-soluble vitamins such as A, D or E. Powders are used for extra potency. Many vitamin C powders contain as much as 4,000 milligrams in a teaspoon. And, for people with allergies, powders have no fillers or binders. Liquids can easily be mixed in beverages for people who have trouble swallowing pills.

Synthetic vitamins might be less likely to upset your budget, but in some individual cases might upset your stomach. Both have produced satisfactory results, but in most cases I recommend natural over synthetic. Synthetic vitamin C, for example, is pure ascorbic acid. Vitamin C from rose hips contains the entire natural complex.

Chelation is also very important. It means the process in which mineral substances are changed into their digestible form. Huge percentages of many non-chelated products will pass through your body without ever being absorbed.

If you use vitamin and mineral supplements, store them in a cool, dark place in a dark container away from direct sunlight. A few kernels of rice at the bottom of a bottle will work as a natural absorbent and guard against moisture.

Vitamins are organic substances and should be consumed with food and minerals for best absorption. The body works on a 24-hour cycle. Your cells don't sleep when you do, nor can they function without continuous oxygen and nutrients. For best results with vitamin and mineral supplements, space them throughout the day and take them after meals. If that's not practical, take half after breakfast and half after dinner. If you must take them all at once, do it after your largest meal.

The range of body functions that can be affected by a vitamin or mineral deficiency is enormous. Be sure to put them high on your list of topics for self-education.

AND A FEW OTHER THINGS

That's a thumbnail look at the six basic nutrients. But there are four other things that should be mentioned here. One of them is good, and Americans don't get enough of it. Three of them are bad, and Americans consume them by the truckload. First the good.

FIBER: This material, which comes from the cell walls of plants, plays a major role in digestion. In recent years we have discovered that it also plays a role in preventing heart disease and colon cancer. Like almost anything involved in publicized nutritional studies, food processors have jumped on the bandwagon with their advertising and labeling. That's OK. Just make sure that any product touted as high in fiber isn't also high in sugar or sodium or fat.

As many as half of all Americans are afflicted with constipation or some form of gastrointestinal distress. Colon cancer is a leading cause of death. Meanwhile, underdeveloped nations whose people eat five to six times as much complex carbohydrates and fiber suffer almost none of either disorder. Like many nutritional choices, the right one is simple and obvious.

Some fiber is water soluble, such as the cellulose in wheat bran and the pectin in apples, citrus fruits and certain vegetables. Other fiber—such as the hemicellulose found in whole grain and other vegetables—absorbs water. Both help promote a smooth and prompt passage through the digestive tract. And both help slow the absorption of glucose into the bloodstream.

A high fiber intake also helps shed excess bodyfat, and may even lower blood pressure.

Eat a wide variety of fresh, whole foods and you'll get plenty of fiber in its various forms. The American Cancer Society recommends 25 to 30 grams a day, but the American average is only 10. Which tells you something about how much fresh, whole food we eat.

SALT: After sugar, sodium chloride is the leading food additive in the United States. Excessive consumption has been linked to depression, bloating, weight gain, kidney disease and, of course, hypertension. The body needs about a quarter of a teaspoon per day. The American average is 20 times that.

Salt—like virtually all tastes—is an acquired one. Talk to people who, usually under doctor's orders, have drastically reduced their sodium intake. They come to *like* the flavor of whole, natural foods. Of course, they have to avoid the lines at the fast-food counter.

Our bodies can't function without their ration of sodium. But a regular diet contains plenty without adding a single grain of salt. Tomatoes and celery, for example, are high in sodium.

The recommended intake is 1,100 to 3,300 milligrams a day. One can of soup contains 900 milligrams, and the stuff is hidden in almost all processed food.

Sweating causes some sodium loss, but under normal conditions body reserves are not depleted even in intense training.

CAFFEINE: This is one powerful legalized drug. Chances are you're not just enjoying your daily coffee and cola, you're addicted to it. Caffeine is intensely psychoactive. It acts directly upon the central nervous system and brings the body an almost immediate sense of clear thought, releases stored sugar from the liver, and gives a feeling of relief from fatigue. That's the "lift" that comes with consuming the big three of caffeine: coffee, colas and chocolate.

The benefits are far outweighed by the risks. The release of stored sugar places heavy stress on the endocrine system. Heavy coffee users often become nervous and jittery. People shifting to decaf sometimes show withdrawal symptoms associated with drug users (and caffeine is a drug).

Some studies suggest that caffeine is linked to prostate problems and benign breast tumors, as well as to bladder cancer. It can rob the body of B complex vitamins, zinc, potassium and other minerals. It contributes to dehydration. It increases acidity in the gastrointestinal tract. Many doctors consider it a culprit in hypertension.

One article in the AMA Journal described a disease called "caffeinism," with symptoms including appetite loss, insomnia, chills, irritability and sometimes a low fever.

A lethal dose of caffeine is about 10 grams. How much are you getting, and where from? Here are a few sources, in milligrams: Coca Cola, 64.7; Dr. Pepper, 60; instant coffee, 66; fresh ground, 146; black tea bags, 46; Anacin, 32 (relieve your headache and get a little boost); Dexetrim, 200 (maybe lose some weight; definitely get a little pep).

Try some substitutes. Ginseng is caffeine-free and gives you a little lift. Herb teas can be invigorating. Club soda or mineral won't give you any caffeine, but you'll be doing your body a big favor.

ALCOHOL: In recent years we've become a lot more conscious of the carnage alcohol causes on our highways. Less dramatically, alcohol abuse causes even more long-term carnage within our bodies. A good argument can be made that alcohol abuse—not crack cocaine—is our greatest drug problem.

Alcohol is not a stimulant; it's a depressant. It does not warm you up; it increases perspiration and loss of body heat. It destroys brain cells by dehydrating them. It depletes the body of numerous vitamins and minerals. Four drinks a day is enough to cause organ damage, to hamper the liver's ability to process fat.

With today's new awareness, you don't need to be told how much bad news lurks in alcoholic beverages of any kind. But it's worth a reminder. Even in moderation, by the way, alcohol is a major negative to athletic performance.

11

Not Weight Loss, But *Fat* Loss

I expect that some readers of this book are obese couch potatoes. I expect that some readers are hard-core weightlifters or marathon runners who, besides their exercise regimen, have adopted a realistic and healthy nutritional lifestyle. I expect that most readers fall somewhere in between. That's a *big* range, and I'm going to have some fitness tips for all of you. Meanwhile, if you're already flat-bellied and if your ideal weight is what you see whenever you step on the scales, then you might want to pass this chapter on to somebody close to you who has a weight problem.

You can't write any kind of fitness book in America without including a chapter on nutrition and weight loss. We are a *fat* country, despite all those slim bodies we see in TV commercials for everything from beer to soda pop to cheeseburgers. The food America eats pretty much guarantees that most of us will be overweight and/or artery-clogged even with a moderate amount of exercise. Take away the exercise and we'd be an *obese* country. The truth is, you can't find many Americans who don't "want to lose some weight."

The key word is "want." How badly do you "want" to lose weight? Maybe you "want" a Mercedes touring car and a tri-level ranch on a hill with a Jacuzzi and an in-ground pool. You don't get those things because they would cost about 100 years of your paycheck. A slim and fit body—which will give you more real pleasure and long-term benefit than all the ranches and Mercedeses in Beverly Hills—doesn't cost a dime. It's there for the taking. So do you "want" it or not?

I've made a decent life out of turning negatives into positives. No way, without the Crohn's and all that agony, was I going to wind up pumping iron and posing my body. Weird, isn't it, how we can be blessed by adversity? Like I said earlier, the beautiful thing about life is that, as long as your mistakes aren't so big that they kill you, life gives you a chance to try again. And that's the way you have to look at an out-of-shape, rundown body. Specifically, in this chapter, a *fat* body. Don't look at it as a prison that you're stuck in; look at it as *a catalyst for change.*

Most people who come to me for nutritional counseling and personal training are seriously overweight. They're not bad people, they're fat people. In fact, I've met some incredibly nice people, some lifelong friends, while doing PT. And the nature of the business pretty much guarantees that my clients are successful people. You don't hire a personal trainer and nutritional consultant unless you're making a dollar or two. Such people almost universally are frustrated beyond belief that they can lead a sales staff to great success, or manage a company, but cannot manage their own bodies. Considering that very few things in life are as important to an individual as the body that he or she must live in, it does say something about the human condition, doesn't it?

People pay me for counseling and training, and then miss sessions. I can't do anything about that. People come up with cockeyed rationales for why they're in the shape they're in—most often, "genetics." More baloney. They don't really "want" to lose weight, and I couldn't do it *for* them if I were their nutrition consultant *and* personal trainer for 10 years.

That's why I give each potential client the rap I outlined in Chapter Nine, the one where I explain it's all up to them. then, before getting on to the nuts and bolts of nutrition and weight loss, I try to explode a number of myths.

MYTH #1: "My mother's fat, my father's fat, I'm fat. It's inherited. I was *born to be fat.*"

FACT: Yes, some people genetically inherit a tendency to form extra fat cells. If they want to be slim, they have to work a little harder at it. But not all basketball players are seven feet tall. And obesity is *not* inherited. Obesity is caused by eating too much fat, skipping meals(!) and forgetting about exercise and stress management. Fat cells then load up with fat and you, as they say, "get fat." Fitness and nutrition will overcome genetics every time. That doesn't necessarily mean that you can look like a fashion model or an NFL wide receiver, but that's not what we're talking about.

MYTH #2: "I can't lose weight because I don't have the discipline to starve myself and ignore hunger."

FACT: This is probably the dumbest of all the myths, because if you are eating the proper foods there is no reason whatsoever to be hungry. You can be "full" and still lose weight. Hunger is your body's way of saying, "Eat." Make yourself artificially hungry and you'll gorge yourself with artificial food. Fad diets and crash diets will rob your body of water or muscle tissue and actually make it easier for your body to accumulate fat. Try fad diets long enough and you could run away and join the circus as Starvini, the Human Yo-Yo.

MYTH #3: "I'm in great shape except my hips, so I'm going to spot reduce."

FACT: You *can't* spot reduce. If you're happy with everything about your body except your waist, or hips, or thighs, or buttocks, then you have to lose fat, period. Your body and your metabolism are symmetrical, even if the mirror tells you otherwise. If you lose weight, you'll lose it throughout your body. Specific exercises can strengthen certain muscles; but that has nothing to do with bodyfat accumulated in the same area. The best overall exercise, by the way, is aerobic—burning excess fat throughout the body by burning calories.

MYTH #4: "I'm not going to think about nutrition to lose weight. I'm going to pick an aerobic exercise—swimming or cycling or running—and I'm going to do it every day. The food part will take care of itself."

FACT: Neither nutrition alone nor exercise alone is the way to lose weight. You have to pay attention to both. The fact is, if you lead an active life—and don't spend hours and hours sitting on the couch—nutrition alone will come closer to doing the job. If you train every day, your body will benefit, no question. But the fact remains that eating 3,500 calories adds a pound and burning 3,500 calories subtracts a pound. You could be an aerobics maniac, but if you pigged out on junk food, you would still become fat. And you cannot exercise away an overdose of cholesterol, or pump iron to reverse the damage that alcohol abuse will do to your liver.

MYTH #5: "I'm not emotionally equipped to lose weight."

FACT: It's scary to include this as one of the five big myths. I'm not a psychologist, and I don't mean this as a slap in the face to that huge crowd of people who desperately want to shed fat but find themselves see-sawing between emotional stress and eating binges. It's a vicious cycle. Gaining fat itself becomes a source of stress, because the victim feels like a failure. But I sincerely believe that, in most cases, this qualifies as a myth. Because I have seen too many cases where a client was able to break out of the trap by *educating* himself or herself, by learning to view food through that second lens. People with emotional problems and stress don't drive up to the self-serve and pump kerosene into their car's gas tank. But, in a manner of speaking, that's exactly what many do to their bodies. Sometimes I think that if everyone knew as much about nutrition as they do about cars—or if they were just as *conscious* of the food they eat as they are about their cars—then the average American would lose five pounds overnight.

Like I said, I'm not a psychologist. But I know from repeated first-hand experience that learning how to make good choices nutritionally by understanding *why* they should be made produces results. And it's not just the waistline that improves. A lot of self-esteem comes along for the ride.

Now for some nuts and bolts.

The first thing to do is to forget about time and forget about your bathroom scales.

You forget about time for three reasons. (1) You didn't get fat overnight and you're not going to get thin overnight. (2) In this diet-crazy country 90 percent of the weight loss schemes you've ever seen or heard of—hundreds or even thousands of them—lie about that simple first fact. So-and-so's quick weight-loss diet. So-and-so's 14-day artichoke plan. Forget it. It's all nonsense. (3) The only time we're talking about is *the rest of your life*. We're not going to switch your car from kerosene to gasoline for a few weeks. This is a permanent switch to the fuel you should have been pumping in the first place.

You forget about the bathroom scales for just one reason. We're not really talking about weight loss—though you probably will lose weight, and certainly will—big-time—if you have a serious weight problem. We're talking about *fat* loss. You want to lose weight fast? It's easy. Dehydrate yourself. That's what a lot of fad diets do. Most of your body is water, so shedding a few pounds quick is a snap. Stupid, but a snap. Or how about muscle? Muscle weighs more than fat, and it's easy to shed muscle. We can sit you on a couch, deprive you of protein, and get rid of some serious pounds in a flash.

Since muscle weighs more than fat—and since you might be adding some muscle from the exercise side of your fitness equation—a moderately overweight person might actually *gain* weight while shedding fat. In any case, I think belt notches and dress sizes are a far more accurate measure of "weight loss" than any bathroom scale. After a month or two on a healthy nutritional regimen, you'll be seeing your progress in the mirror instead of looking at a couple of ticks on a scale that might mean nothing except that there's a little less water in your body today.

Next comes the old—and highly controversial—question, "How much should I weigh?" There's no absolute answer, and no easy answer—except that you probably should weigh less. One study at Harvard Medical School suggests that even moderate overweight is more harmful than generally believed. In fact, people weighing at least 10 percent below average for their frame showed the lowest death rates. Another study by the National Institutes for Health showed the same results—as long as the below-average weight was not a result of illness, of course.

If you want to seriously pursue this business of how much you should weigh, you'll have to spend a lot of money. Because what you really want to find out is your desirable bodyfat level, and the only precisely accurate way to measure it is at a high-tech testing center, using an underwater weighing method. That's not real practical. Second-best is through skin caliper measurements—but only when tested by a skilled professional, and that will cost money, too.

If you're not scared off by arithmetic, you can estimate your own body mass index (BMI). It's not highly accurate, but it's free. Here's what you do to calculate your BMI:

(1) Convert your weight into kilograms by dividing your weight (without clothes) in pounds by 2.2.

(2) Convert your height in inches to meters by dividing your height (without shoes) by 39.4; then square that number (multiply it by itself).

(3) Divide your weight in kilograms by your height in meters. That number is an approximation of your body mass index.

As an example, take a man who is 5-foot-10 and weighs 160. Divide 160 pounds by 2.2 to get 72.72 kilograms. Divide 70 inches by 39.4 to get 1.78 meters. Square 1.78 to get 3.168. Then divide 72.72 by 3.168 and you have a body mass index of 22.95.

For women with average musculature, a BMI above 23 often indicates overweight. For men, it's a reading above 24. Obesity (20 percent above the normal range) begins at 27.2 for men and 26.9 for women.

That's all pretty complicated and not very accurate. I still think that well-toned muscles, a strong heart, and an ability to look in a mirror without flinching are the truly meaningful measures of a body's fitness.

Traditionally, the measurements that launch any weight-loss program are the weight-for-age-and-sex charts and the calorie charts. People check out the weight chart, then start counting calories and stepping anxiously on the scales. My own view is that if losing bodyfat were as simple as counting calories, then shedding blubber would be as easy as skipping breakfast. A lot of people do just that, and fail. Isn't it interesting that somebody would answer the truism that "You are what you eat" by eating nothing at all?

Two variables really determine what you are going to weigh:

(1) Your energy balance—the number of calories you consume each day (input), compared with the number of calories you burn (output).

(2) Your body composition—your percentage of bodyfat compared with lean tissue.

That's because your energy output depends on your basal metabolism rate (BMR), the rate at which you burn calories while at rest. And *lean tissue is more active than fat tissue in burning calories.*

Obviously, exercise is a key part of this picture. Anaerobic exercise builds lean tissue. And aerobic exercise will raise your BMR for hours after you are through exercising—meaning you'll still be burning calories. Nutritionally speaking, there is one humongous fact about nutrition and BMR that blows away all the old wive's tales about "dieting."

Spacing your caloric intake throughout the day—throwing away the "eat three square meals by the clock" tradition and eating five or six meals a day—will *raise your basal metabolism rate.* Your body's fat-burning activity will be elevated for almost all your waking hours. The hormonal signals that cause fat cells to multiply will be reduced. In other words, here's yet another reason to think less about how much you eat and more about *what* and when you eat.

The main thing is cutting down on dietary fat—the vast majority of which finds a home under your skin and becomes the "weight" that you really want to lose. Remember also that the body can utilize protein only in relatively small, rationed quantities. And that simple carbohydrates are cheap, junky fuel good for a quick high and a quick crash—and for conversion to fat if consumed in excess. Where does that leave you in the search for your best dietary friend? Right. Complex carbohydrates.

Complex carbos are certainly your metabolism's best friend, when it comes to bodyfat. In scientific terms, complex carbos are vermagenic and fats are non-vermagenic. In other words, carbohydrates generate much more heat—burn more energy—per calorie. Since dietary fat already *is* fat, it takes very little energy—about three calories—to convert dietary fat into new bodyfat. It takes about 23 calories to turn 100 calories of carbohydrate into fat. Since complex carbohydrates (and many fruits and vegetables) generally are rich in fiber, they are absorbed more slowly, contributing to a satisfied feeling. They also require more energy to digest.

All of which suggests that you can't possibly do better than getting into a close, familiar relationship with pastas, baked potatoes, whole-grain breads and rolls and bagels—some of the very foods that the fad diets would have you ignore.

My nutritional consulting clients almost invariably assure me that they eat a wide variety of food. Usually it turns out to be a wide variety of fat-drenched foods and an excess of protein and simple, empty carbohydrates. One way to replace the sense of food deprivation, real or imagined, is to take a real run at the enormous variety of fruits, vegetables and pastas that you probably don't try very often. Use new herbs and spices as replacements for the fats that you remove from your diet, and to stimulate the taste buds.

High-quality nutrients in vegetables, legumes, whole grains, fruits, fish, poultry and non-fat dairy products make it easy to keep a lid on calorie intake without getting into calorie-counting mania. I strongly recommend against any "diet" that aims to drastically reduce calories, such as the under-1,200 calorie diets that are popular in some circles. If you go that route, do it only under the guidance of a doctor. If you choose to limit yourself to 1,200 to 1,800 calories a day, make sure that you are getting a reasonably accurate count. The best guide is *Calories and Your Weight,* available from the U.S. Government Printing Office. This being the '90s, calorie-counting software can also be purchased for your home or office computer.

A gram scale for your kitchen isn't a bad idea for keeping track of fat- or protein-dense foods such as meat and poultry. After a while you'll be able to eyeball a piece of meat fairly accurately. But at first, you won't believe your eyes. It doesn't take much meat to cross the line from protein consumption to fat production.

You'll also do well to sort out the difference between "hunger" and "appetite." Hunger is an unpleasant physical sensation caused by an urgent need for food. Appetite is a desire to eat whether or not you are hungry. Your appetite might need discipline, but you should never be hungry. Remember that appetite is affected by habits, social situations and emotional pressures. In the early stages of your new nutritional regimen, you might have to plan strategy just like someone who is shaking the nicotine habit—avoiding situations that trigger your addiction.

Make a production out of quality instead of quantity. Put on some music, get out the tablecloth, relearn how to have conversation while you're dining, instead of just stuffing your mouth.

You've heard a million times that you should relax and eat more slowly. Why? Partly it's to give your digestive system a break, instead of forcing it to treat every meal like an emergency rush job. But another reason is that it will take less food to leave you feeling satisfied and "full." There are hormonal reasons for this, and suffice it to say that it takes about 20 minutes for the insulin in your cerebral spinal fluid to send a "full" message to the brain. You can eat a reasonable amount of food in 20 minutes and be full. Or you can eat like a demented hog for 20 minutes and be full. Your choice.

That little scenario is complicated for obese people, whose insulin generally enters the bloodstream more slowly—meaning it takes them longer to be satisfied. Take smaller bites. Pause longer between bites. Take *control.*

Empty the house of junk food. You're not going to be eating it any more, and you won't be doing friends and loved ones any favors by feeding it to them. One good way to come up with new dishes and snack recipes that will keep *you* happy is to scour the cookbooks, and your own imagination, for recipes that will please *them.*

Drink lots of water between meals. And remember that even though you're probably going to be eating more often under your new regimen, just before going to bed is *not* one of those times. An evening snack of a bagel, or a frozen banana, or a pasta salad is fine—as long as it's a few hours before bedtime.

Try keeping a diary of what you eat and drink. Memory won't cut it when you want to reconstruct a picture of a day's, or a week's, nutrition.

The bottom line is that we're talking about behavioral change, and your *feelings* about food. Just as with your behavior and attitudes in any area, there is no substitute for education. You don't tend a garden or maintain a car or learn to play piano on impulse. You learn and you practice. You care about what you are doing and you pay close, regular attention to it. Where your body is concerned, you can never learn too many why's and how's. They will help you keep viewing a plate of food through that second, analytical lens.

Mood swings and stress are real enough. Try, for starters, to channel them somewhere besides your mouth. I assume you don't come home and kick the cat. That's good. Now start thinking about the fact that you shouldn't come home and eat a quart of ice cream, either.

This is one of several areas where exercise becomes a super partner to nutrition in weight loss. Instead of taking it out on that quart of ice cream, take it out in a long brisk walk, or a jog, or a tennis game, or a swim—or whatever exercise fits your taste and your current body condition.

Frustration, boredom, a loss of motivation—these kinds of emotional swings occur to all of us. We get stalled by mental blocs and psychological factors that I'm not qualified to analyze. But I do know that we have to prevent them from slopping over into what happens to our bodies. And that if you arrive at one of those negative plateaus, it is vital that you take immediate constructive action.

Often I'll choose a new form of exercise, or an increased level of activity. That'll boost my metabolism, and help fight boredom. (If you're not a weightlifter, believe me there are times when all those reps *do* get boring.) I also try to add something new to my diet. Any change of pace—expanding your social network, meeting a new friend, becoming more involved in a project or a hobby—can help get your goal-orientation back on track.

Rewards are important. Sometimes we forget how often we reward ourselves with food. So it'll help immensely if you consciously replace hot fudge sundaes and pizzas with non-edible rewards. Get out to a movie. Get out to the bookstore and buy a new book to read for pleasure. (Load up on nutrition books, but avoid any that include phrases like "14 Days," "Easy" or "Miracle.") Buy earrings. Go to a concert. Get a new CD and enjoy. *Bon appetit* doesn't have to mean food.

12

Fueling for Performance

Nutrition and exercise go hand in hand. But the picture is more complicated than a high five after a big play. A better analogy might be an integrated circuit from your TV set. A bad analogy definitely would be the "one candy bar equals one winning drive to the basket" that you see in TV commercials. Physical performance is all about energy, but it's *not* about mainlining candy bars to win the NBA playoffs.

Muscles use energy. The more you use your muscles, the more energy they consume. Sustained exercise of your most important muscle—your heart—will use even more energy. That's why aerobic exercise—putting your heart and lungs into overdrive, fanning the calorie-burning flames with oxygen—will help you trim your body. Assuming, of course, that you're eating right.

Your body can get fuel for exercise from several sources. The main source, the master fuel, is complex carbohydrates. The digestive system turns carbos into glucose. When this blood sugar is transported to a muscle, it becomes glycogen and is stored there for energy—about 90 minutes' worth. Different kinds of exercise—at different levels of intensity and duration—determine how much energy you use, how quickly you use it, and whether you are burning muscle glycogen, blood glucose, or two secondary sources of energy.

One of these secondary sources (good news) is fat. Depending on the kind of exercise you are performing, exercise *can* burn up fat.

The other source (bad news) is protein. If your body is burning protein for fuel, that means two things: (1) you are extremely fatigued, and (2) your body is feeding on itself.

Anaerobic exercise is an intense thrust of energy for a matter of 10 to 15 seconds. Traditional weightlifting exercises are anaerobic. Those heavy, quick bursts with the weights build and strengthen muscle, but the anaerobic pathway allows muscles to utilize only one kind of energy: muscle glycogen.

Aerobic exercise elevates the heart rate and sustains it. Generally, it takes 15 or 20 minutes of exercise to get your cardiovascular system up to speed. We're all familiar by now with gym-based "aerobics classes." All those ladies jumping and twisting to old Boz Skaggs music are actually burning glucose 18 to 19 times faster than the dude in the next room doing 10 quick presses with a 200-pound barbell. And, as you'll see in a moment, the aerobic stompers can actually burn up fat—*as long as they don't get too intense in their workout!*

Cross-training, a combination of both aerobic and anaerobic exercise, builds strength *and* endurance. This is a golden pathway to fitness through exercise, and we'll talk about it extensively in Part Three.

Low to moderate exercise—up to 60 percent of cardiovascular capacity—can be fueled almost entirely through the aerobic pathway. Hormonal changes and decreased insulin output promote the release of fatty acids from fat tissue into the bloodstream. These fatty acids, combined with fat pools in muscle tissue, supply about half the energy for low to moderate exercise. Muscle glycogen and blood glucose supply the rest.

During high intensity exercise—70 percent or more of aerobic capacity—the body does not use fat as fuel. Fat simply can't supply energy fast enough for high intensity exercise, with the body straining to supply enough oxygen to match its workload. Glucose delivers about five calories per liter of oxygen, and fat delivers only 4.65 calories, so the body shifts to glucose and glycogen as an energy source. The accumulation of lactic acid is another reason for the shift. Lactic acid, a waste product of high intensity exercise, hinders mobilization of fatty acids from adipose (fat) tissue.

Duration of exercise also plays a major role in whether or not you burn up any fat in the gym or on the road. Muscle glycogen is the predominant fuel for the first 30 to 60 minutes of most types of exercise. It takes that long for fatty acids to be freed for use as fuel. The longer you exercise, the greater the contribution of fat tissue to your energy consumption. If you exercise moderately for four to six hours, fat can contribute as much as 70 percent of the calories you burn. The longer you exercise, the less intense it must be.

The basic nutritional message here? If you're a skinny marathoner, you'll want to consume great quantities of the master fuel—complex carbos—before hitting the road. Your muscles will be in glycogen heaven. But if burning up fat is one reason you're about to step on a treadmill, you're not interested in blocking or delaying your body's switch to fat as a fuel. The pre-workout dose of complex carbo energy is not the proper strategy for a weight-loser.

Ironically, the more fit you are, the easier it is for your body to burn fat. Nobody ever said life was fair. The scientific proof is this: Endurance training increases an athlete's ability to perform more aerobically during exactly the same exercise. In other words, to use more fat and less glycogen. When I said the body starts to accumulate lactic acid at about 70 percent of aerobic capacity, I was referring to people well along in a fitness regimen—individuals in training. For an untrained, out-of-shape person, lactic acid starts to accumulate at about 50 percent of aerobic capacity.

This point at which the lactic acid starts building up is called the anaerobic threshold. Increase your anaerobic threshold and you'll increase your ability to burn up fat instead of glycogen. Obviously, your athletic performance in any kind of sustained event will also improve greatly. And there's a double bonus. Trained (fit) individuals also can store about $1^1/_2$ times as much glycogen in their muscle tissue. So they have more glycogen to begin with, and will burn it up at a slower rate.

None of this means that an athlete should eat a high-fat diet. Even the leanest marathoner stores more bodyfat than he or she will ever need during exercise. If you're dieting, you have probably figured out by now that your new nutritional lifestyle (high in complex carbos) means you will be burning a lot of glycogen. Right. Your goal is to increase the use of fat as fuel through endurance training, not by eating fat. Couch potatoes who eat fatty foods cut back their carbo intake, which decreases muscle glycogen, which reduces ability to sustain exercise, which stops you from getting to the point where you burn up fat.

CARBOHYDRATES AND PERFORMANCE

Stores of muscle glycogen begin to reach low levels in high intensity exercise that exceeds 90 minutes. When glycogen reaches a critically low supply, the body leaves the athlete two choices: slow the pace dramatically, or collapse from exhaustion.

Glycogen can also be depleted in a slow process over several days of repeated heavy training, when you do not eat enough complex carbohydrates to replace what you've used. When this happens, glycogen stores drop each day—and the athlete wonders why he's not able to maintain his training intensity. That's often the explanation for a "stale" feeling in an exercise program. Instead of the "overtraining" that often gets blamed, it's an insufficiency of complex carbos—and sometimes dehydration.

(To be specific, if you're in advanced training, we're comparing a 40 percent carbo diet [300–350 grams] with a 70 percent carbo diet [500–600 grams] during repeated days of two-hour workouts.)

In one study, fit athletes who started out like gangbusters on an intensive training program were not able to perform even moderate level exercise after seven days on a low-carbo diet—with muscle glycogen stores dropping each day.

"Training glycogen depletion," to use the textbook phrase, happens to athletes involved in exercise other than endurance training in the gym. Football, basketball and soccer players—any athlete who uses repeated near-maximum bursts of effort—can experience the same type of exhaustion. Telltale signs are inability to maintain normal exercise intensity and a sudden weight loss of several pounds. Lack of carbos, and lack of rest days, are culprits.

If you are in serious training, you should be eating a diet rich in complex carbos and you should be taking periodic rest days, during which your muscles will replenish their stores of glycogen. I preach this so much that you'd think the Complex Carbo Sales Board was paying me off. But the imbalance between fats and complex carbos is our single biggest nutritional failing. For athletes, it's especially important. The average American diet gets 42 percent of calories from carbohydrates. It should be 60 percent. For athletes who are exercising strenuously for several hours daily (or for people who do hard physical labor for a living), it should be 70 percent. Now you know why.

And one more word about simple vs. complex carbos. Yes, simple carbos also provide glycogen synthesis. But complex carbos provide more nutrition—including fiber, iron and B complex vitamins necessary for metabolism. Most importantly, complex carbos are time-released, and will not turn to fat if not burned up immediately. My own recommendation is a non-training diet of 60 percent carbohydrates—of which 10 percent can be simple carbos from fruits and juices.

CARBOHYDRATE OVERLOADING

That's not a negative phrase. It refers to an athletic strategy for nearly doubling muscle glycogen storage before an event. Obviously, the greater the pre-exercise glycogen content of the muscle, the greater the endurance potential. Even if you're not a competitive athlete, you'll probably find the nuts and bolts of the strategy interesting.

There's an old way and a new way.

The old way—which I tried for a time myself—was basically an exhaustive weeklong training regimen, followed by a precise exercise and nutrition regimen for the last six days before an event. For the first three days of the last six, the athlete would consume a *low*-carbohydrate diet while continuing to work out, thus lowering muscle glycogen storage even further. Then, the last three days before the event, the athlete would rest and consume a *high*-complex carbo diet to promote muscle glycogen storage and super compensation for the depleted stores. During those last three days, you would consume about 100 calories of complex carbos per hour.

For many years, this was considered the optimal way to achieve maximum glycogen storage. But it had some serious drawbacks. For one thing, you could develop hypoglycemia (low blood sugar) while starving yourself of carbos. You could also develop ketosis (increased blood acids), with side effects like nausea, fatigue, dizziness, diarrhea and irritability. Live and learn. Like I said, I was my own guinea pig from the day I came out of the hospital. Many of the things I've learned came the hard way.

The new and improved version of carbo loading makes sense, and it provides muscle glycogen stores equal to the old, disproved method.

Six days before competition the athlete exercises strenuously, to 70 or 75 percent of aerobic capacity, for 90 minutes. On that day, and for the next two days, he or she consumes a normal diet of 50 percent carbohydrates—about 350 grams a day. On the second and third day, the training is decreased to 40 minutes. For the next two days the athlete eats a high complex carbohydrate diet (about 70 percent, or 550 grams) and reduces training to 20 minutes at 70 percent of aerobic capacity. On the last day, the athlete rests while maintaining a high complex carbo diet.

This modified loading method allows you to maintain high intensity training longer, but will not affect pace for the first hour of your event. Runners who used the loading method for one 30K event doubled their glycogen levels. Both groups "ran their race" for the first hour, but the carbo-loaded group was able to stay on a faster pace longer in the latter stages of the race.

The old-time carbo loading method used a carbo starvation period because it was thought necessary to trigger maximum levels of glycogen storage. Now we know better—that *endurance training* is the primary stimulus for muscle glycogen production and storage. The exercise to deplete storage, by the way, must be the same exercise as the event that you are preparing for. That's because glycogen is depleted—and manufactured and stored—in the muscles you use. So a runner, for example, needs to deplete storage by running, rather than by cycling.

In the final three days, when the athlete tapers training activity, he needs a high complex carbo diet because these are the real "loading" days of the regimen. That's why it's essential to reduce training during this period. Otherwise, you'll use too much of the stored glycogen and defeat the whole scheme.

If you have difficulty downing all that pasta and such, commercial carbohydrate supplements are available. And if you have diabetes or high triglycerides, loading can lead to medical complications. Check with your doctor before trying the regimen.

Each gram of glycogen you store also means that you're storing water. Some athletes report feelings of stiffness or heaviness as a result. In bodybuilding, that's just fine—because muscle is 75 percent water. The more glycogen you store, the more your muscles will fill with fluid and the more they're going to look "ripped" or "cut"—well-defined. Remember, you won't have this water between skin and muscle; you'll have it *in* your muscle.

CARBO INTAKE BEFORE EXERCISING

While you are exercising or performing athletically, the body relies on pre-existing glycogen or fat storage for energy. A pre-exercise meal or snack won't do anything for you immediately, but the carbohydrates can add to blood glucose—and energy—if you exercise for more than an hour. That's why athletes who compete in a prolonged endurance event that relies heavily on blood sugar won't perform as well if they skip breakfast. The overnight fast lowers their liver glycogen storage, the main source of blood sugar.

In the past, athletes have been discouraged from eating on the morning before training or a competition. Common advice is to eat two to three hours before exercising, so if there's a morning track meet or an early appointment at the gym, most people will skip breakfast. The rationale is that any food remaining in the stomach at the start of exercise might nauseate you when blood is diverted from the gastrointestinal tract to the exercising muscle. Athletes also have been advised to avoid high-carbohydrate meals immediately before training, on grounds that higher insulin levels might cause hypoglycemia or fatigue. Actually, there is a great range of personal reaction here. Some athletes in endurance training are insensitive to lowered blood sugars. (I'm one of them.) There's really no substitute for experimenting with your own body's reaction to pre-exercise meals.

The simple fact is that carbo feeding before exercise can help restore depleted liver and muscle glycogen storage. If gastric emptying is a concern, then you can always try a commercial liquid meal. They're high in carbo calories, contribute to hydration, and can be consumed nearer to the time of a competition because of the shorter gastric emptying time. They may help *prevent* pre-event nausea in a tense athlete. Liquid meals also are more convenient during daylong competitions, such as track meets or triathlons or tennis tournaments.

How much carbohydrates should an athlete eat before an event? The consensus suggests one to four grams per kilogram of bodyweight, consumed one to four hours before exercising. To prevent possible gastro distress, decrease the intake if you eat nearer to the time of the event—four grams per kilo of bodyweight four hours prior to the event, down to one gram one hour prior to the event.

Good examples of pre-exercise carbo foods: breads (adding some jam or jelly), fruits, juices and non-fat yogurt.

What about consuming simple sugar before exercise? Studies on the subject are all over the map. For sure, consuming a candy bar before anaerobic exercise—such as weight training—will not increase performance because your body already has plenty of glycogen stored for the activity. It could be useful, however, for a long-distance runner who will need energy when muscle glycogen falls to a low level. Again, there are great individual differences here. You should test your own reaction in training.

FLUID INTAKE BEFORE EXERCISE

For peak performance, you should be fully hydrated before training or competing. Drink 16 to 20 ounces of water through the two hours before training, and drink another 16 ounces of cold fluid 10 to 15 minutes before starting.

Drinking the full quota of fluids just before exercise can produce hyperhydration. Some people think hyperhydrating improves thermoregulation by shortening the usual delay in sweating and decreasing the quantity of sweat. No serious advantages have been proven for this strategy, however. Particularly in hot weather, I'd suggest an

Suspension wires were strung for the Verrazano Narrows Bridge but the traffic deck wasn't hung yet when Dad first took me to see it. The water, and the view from Manhattan to infinity, became very special to me a few years later.

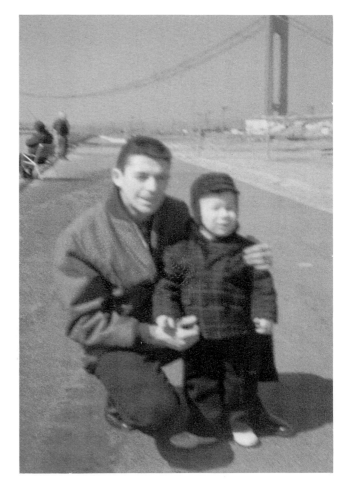

Dad and I had some of our best times hunting and fishing. And he made an urban cowboy out of me (below left) at a very young age. That's my first bike (below right), complete with training wheels. Before long, the training wheels would be gone and I'd be pedaling down to Shore Road to see the bridge and the water.

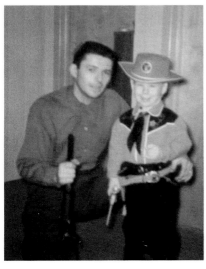

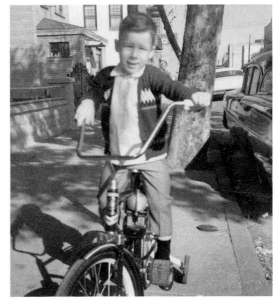

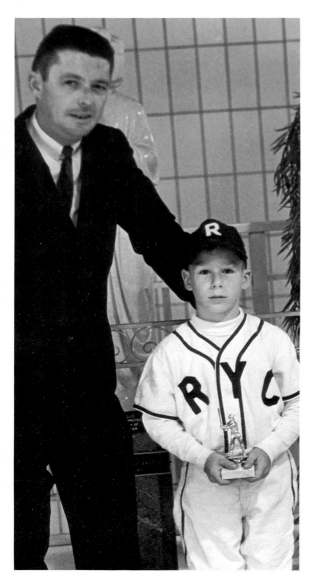

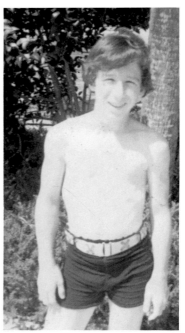

That's a studio portrait (below) at age 4½. I was scrawny, and always getting sick on birthdays and special occasions. We all thought "that's just the way Peter is." Then we learned about Crohn's disease. Soon after I came out of the hospital, Mom and Dad took me to Florida (above). A good wind would have blown me into the ocean. I weighed 86 pounds.

The uniform letters stand for Regina Youth Center. I put the "Peewee" in Peewee League. Dad was proud of the trophy. I guess I was, too, though I look more like amazed.

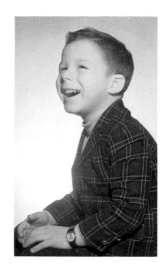

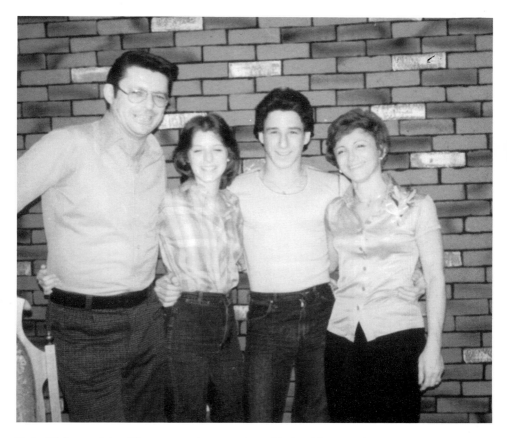

Pete Nielsen, sister Kim, me and my mother, Marie. After my Crohn's was diagnosed, everybody in the family blamed themselves for the incredible tension in the house where this frail kid (me) lived. We were all wrong.

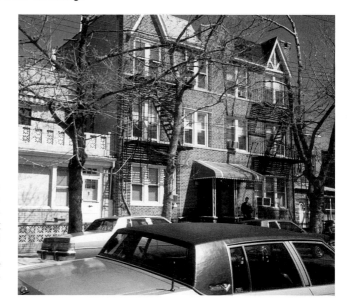

My grandmother's apartment building on Sixty-Seventh Street in Brooklyn. Actually, she owns the right half of the building (and still lives on the first floor). Mom and Kim live on the second floor, in the apartment where I grew up.

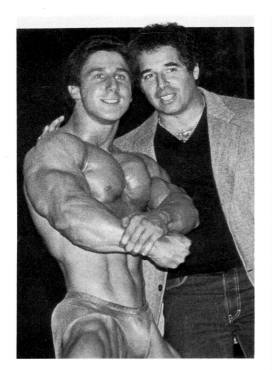

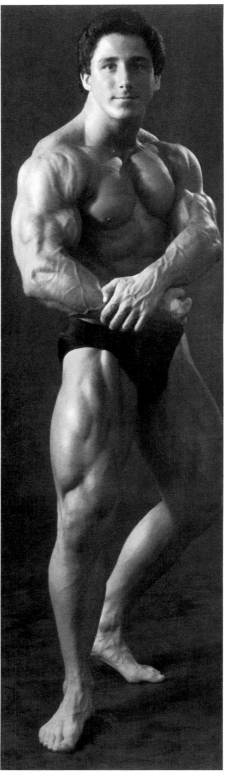

Julie Levine (with me above at the Mr. New York contest) taught me how to be a bodybuilder. The shot at right is my look when I won the Teenage Eastern America, and my Dad shocked me by joining me on stage for the award. The trophy below was my very first—fifth place in Armstrong County, Pa. My Dad drove for hours to get me there. We buried the trophy with him.

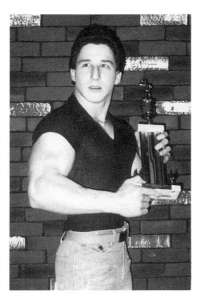

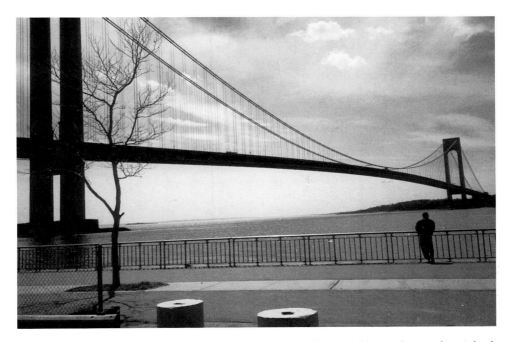

Revisiting Shore Road in 1990. My whole life changed one cold morning as I watched dawn come up over the bridge. To this day, the waterfront panorama at the end of Brooklyn is still a big-time reality check for me.

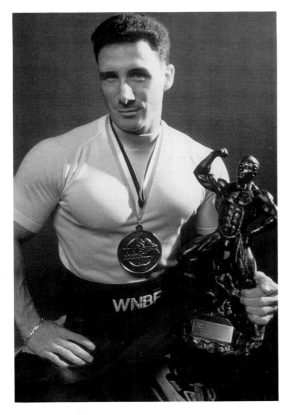

Skip ahead to 1992. This is my current look—a lot more mellow, I hope. Bodybuilding is just a part of my life, but you can't help loving those trophies. The medal is for finishing fourth in the World Cup after coming out of retirement in November 1991. The trophy is for taking first place in the NGA regional USA a month earlier. Young dudes don't get to have all the fun.

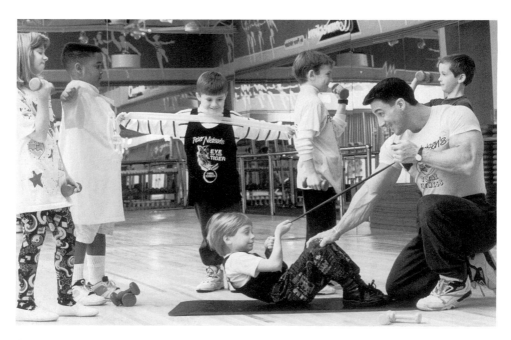

I make a good part of my living helping middle-aged people get back into shape. But kids are at the heart of my message. In the TV era, we've made a horror story out of childhood nutrition and exercise. The very best thing you can do for your kids is put them on a healthy pathway.

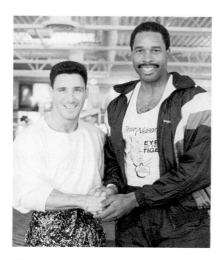

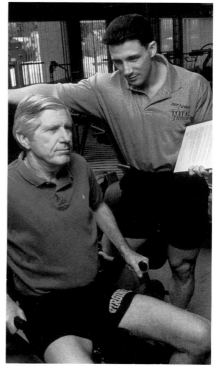

"PT" means physical therapy (right) as well as personal training. Many of my clients—burdened by neuromuscular disease—have discovered their best hope in the gym. Pro athletes often drop by when they're in town. I want to remind you that Dave Winfield (above) is closer to 7 feet tall than 6.

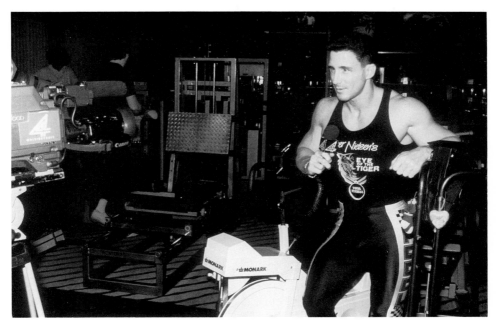

That's me in front of a Channel 4 camera at the gym. TV is fun, and it reaches more people than you can reach in a thousand speeches. Most people watch from a couch, but my segment gives me a chance to pull them off the couch and into action.

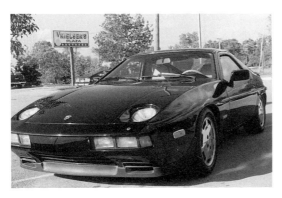

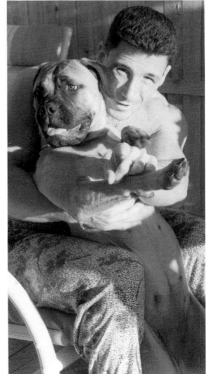

Two animals I love: my Porsche 928, which is no longer really me, and which I hide in the garage most of the time; and Angel, my gentle bull mastiff. The Porsche was only an extravagance. Angel is a friend.

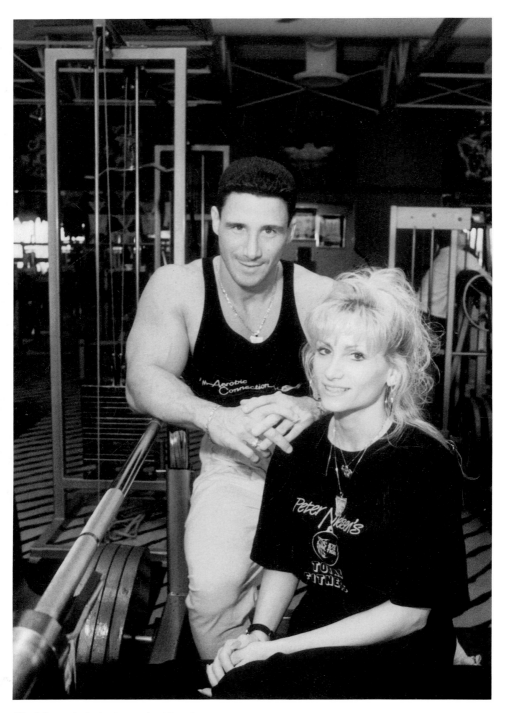

Cindy's a whole lot better looking than me, so we decided to make this picture bigger. She's no slouch in the gym herself. Cindy has her own personal training clientele, and she can outrun me by several miles. Best of all, she never complains about broiling chicken breasts twice a day.

athlete should drink no more fluid—probably about 20 ounces—than he or she will be comfortable with.

What kind of fluid? More than 15 minutes before exercising, stick with water. In the final 15 minutes, water-diluted fruit juice or a sports drink is a good choice if the activity will be longer than an hour.

I shouldn't have to tell you that caffeine is a lousy pre-exercise beverage.

FLUID INTAKE DURING EXERCISE

Individual responses vary tremendously. Drinking fluids during exercise is as much an art as a science, even though there are tons of reports on the subject. In any case, fluid replacement during exercise—training or competition—is vital to prevent thermal damage. In training, it helps you get into a routine for drinking fluids during competition.

You should aim to replace at least 50 percent of fluid loss while you exercise. Drink four to six ounces of cold fluid (40 to 50 degrees) every 10 to 15 minutes. Cold fluid will not only help cool the core body temperature, but will leave the stomach more rapidly than warm fluid. Warmer fluids make sense if you're exercising in cool or cold weather.

The idea is to replace lost fluids, so one of the prime attributes in choosing a drink is that you find it palatable. If you like it, you'll drink it. Water is palatable to most anyone. Water also is inexpensive and easily absorbed. Good stuff, that water.

Sports drinks combine glucose and sodium to promote rapid absorption from the small intestine. That's OK. Just remember that any benefits of carbo replacement are strictly limited to endurance activities. If you drink juice, it should be diluted at least by half.

CARBOHYDRATES AFTER EXERCISE

You know that eating a high carbohydrate diet during intensive training is vital to replenish muscle glycogen stores. The time period when you eat after exercise is also important. The sooner the better.

The only serious study I've found on the subject measured muscle glycogen production when two grams of carbohydrates per kilogram of bodyweight were consumed immediately after exercise, two hours after exercise, and four hours after exercise. Two hours after exercise, glycogen production was cut by a third. Four hours after exercise it was cut by 45 percent.

There are several possible explanations. Blood flow to the muscle is greater immediately after exercise. Muscle cell is more receptive to glycogen. And the cells are more sensitive to insulin, which promotes glycogen production.

Commercial complex carbo drinks can make sense here, because many athletes are not hungry for a meal after heavy exercise.

How much should you consume after heavy exercise? The best evidence suggests about 400 calories (or 100 grams) of carbos within 15 minutes of a workout.

FLUID INTAKE AFTER EXERCISE

Intensive exercise blunts the sensation of thirst, and it will be quenched before you replace the fluids you have lost in a workout or competition. That's why you're got to be deliberate about fluid replacement after your event or workout. For every pound of bodyweight lost, you should drink about 16 ounces of liquid. Start drinking as soon as the workout is over—even before you shower—and then keep drinking at a comfortable pace.

The temperature of what you drink is less important at this point, but a warm drink can prevent hypothermia on a cold day of outdoor activity.

If you undertake moderate exercise in moderate temperature, you're going to lose more water than electrolytes—meaning water is the crucial nutrient to replace. Plain water is fine. A sweet-tasting fluid has only the side benefit of stimulating you to drink more. Alcohol or caffeine—in coffee or in soda pop—are diuretics, and will only make you lose more water.

Fluid replacement generally follows the same principles no matter what your activity, but some sports need special consideration. Fluid should never be restricted for football players, for example. In hot weather, exercising underneath all that gear can generate incredible fluid loss. Endurance runners and cyclists must drink fluid while running or pedaling. Protecting against dehydration is such an important factor that runners and cyclists must learn to function with fluid in their stomachs, even if it's a personal discomfort. Swimmers—who bury themselves in water—lose pounds of the stuff while sitting around in the sunshine between events.

In some quarters, two particular sports raise fluid deprivation to a near-criminal level. Boxing and wrestling are based on weight classifications, and the easiest way to make weight is to shed water. It's dangerous and stupid.

Water plays a key role in athletic performance by maintaining blood volume, necessary for cardiovascular function and for regulating body temperature. Thirst is an unreliable barometer of your hydration. That's why athletes—and recreational competitors—should follow the guidelines above.

Fluid replacement is even more important with the very young and the very old.

Children have lower heat tolerance—a lower sweating capacity, and a lower cardiac output, which makes it harder to dissipate excess body heat. In cold temperatures, their extremities are more likely to freeze. Kids should drink 10 to 14 ounces of fluid before going out to play. I know it sounds impractical, but a boy or girl playing in warm temperatures should continue to replace fluids at the rate of about three ounces every 10 to 15 minutes during activity.

As for older people, one survey found that after 24 hours of fluid deprivation, 67- to 75-year-old men were less thirsty and drank less water than 20- to 31-year-old men. Besides which, many older people are taking many medications—often including diuretics. Fluid consumption needs to be carefully monitored as we grow older.

13

The Building Block to Muscle

Protein is the royalty of nutrients. It is found in some of our highest-priced foods. (It's also found in some of our lowest-priced foods, but they tend to get snubbed—as if you couldn't possibly find a *protein* living at that address.) Many people eat unhealthy meals every day, confident they are doing themselves a favor because they are loading up on protein. It is, after all, the stuff that builds muscle.

Several generations were raised on nutritional folklore that went something like, "Protein is real food; the rest of it is junk and fattening."

The fact is, protein *is* the royalty of nutrients, but to have a healthy relationship with protein you must treat it like royalty: Protein has a very limited schedule, and you must accommodate it. If you are building muscle, through weightlifting or otherwise, you absolutely must take a scientific approach to protein consumption. Otherwise, you will be tearing yourself apart when you think you are building yourself up.

Anaerobic exercise *breaks down* muscle tissue. Your musculature then replaces itself with larger, stronger tissue—*if* you are consuming the proper amount of protein *at the right time*. Since the body can utilize just 35 to 40 grams of protein in any 2½-hour period, sitting down and gorging yourself on protein will produce nothing but fat and toxic wastes. So the amount of protein you consume through the day must be carefully adjusted to fit your exercise regimen. The more muscle you tear down, the more protein you need to replace it. The less you exercise, the more you need a common-sense diet of complex carbohydrates.

This protein connection also often explains why crash diets fail—or even boomerang, leaving the puzzled dieter weighing more than he or she did in the first place. A tremendous lowering of calorie intake for an extended period lowers the basal metabolism rate (BMR), making it difficult if not impossible to continue shedding body fat. If you foolishly go on a starvation diet while exercising, and deprive yourself of protein, you will *lose muscle* instead of fat.

While in training it is absolutely essential that you eat *four, five or even six meals* a day—not just for the other nutritional benefits of that regimen that we have talked about, but to get protein to your muscles. If you eat more than 40 grams of protein in any $2^1/_2$-hour period, you might as well be pouring the precious stuff out on your driveway.

So what's an accurate, practical way of selecting and monitoring your protein intake? How much protein is enough?

You'll read advice ranging from one-half gram of protein to a full gram of protein per pound of body weight—a 100 percent variance!

The chart at the end of this chapter—multiplying your ideal body weight by your activity load—tells what's right for you.

I use exactly the same formula. Because I'm a bodybuilder in training, because I do a tremendous amount of intense anaerobic exercise, I need a large amount of protein. The way I get it is by eating six carefully planned meals a day, none of which look like anything out of a Norman Rockwell Thanksgiving scene. (You'll see a daily menu example in the next chapter.) This is the *only* way I can get the protein I need. It *must* be spaced through the day.

If you're a weightlifter, or training intensively in another sport, you can follow my program out the window and benefit greatly. If you exercise moderately, or lightly, or not at all, this will strike you as one bizarre-looking regimen. But remember, my goal here is not to get every reader eating chicken breasts three or four times a day. It's for you to understand how the body accepts protein, and how you must incorporate that into your own nutrition regimen—whatever your physical workload.

How to Determine
Daily Protein Requirement

GRAMS OF PROTEIN PER DAY, DEPENDING ON ACTIVITY LEVEL
(Multiply by ideal body weight, using chart below.)

.5 grams per lb.: Sedentary, no sports or fitness training
.6 grams per lb: Jogger or in light fitness training
.7 grams per lb: Sports participant or moderate training three days a week
.8 grams per lb: Moderate training every day, aerobic or weights
.9 grams per lb: Heavy weight training daily
1.0 grams per lb: Heavy weight training daily plus sports training, or two-a-day weight training

Ideal Body Weight	Total Daily Protein Grams					
	.5	.6	.7	.8	.9	1.0
90	45	54	63	72	81	90
100	50	60	70	80	90	100
110	55	66	77	88	99	110
120	60	72	84	96	108	120
130	65	78	91	104	117	130
140	70	84	98	112	126	140
150	75	90	105	120	135	150
160	80	96	112	128	144	160
170	85	102	119	136	153	170
180	90	108	126	144	162	180
190	95	114	133	152	171	190
200	100	120	140	160	180	200
210	105	126	147	168	189	210
220	110	132	154	176	198	220
230	115	130	161	184	207	230
240	120	144	168	192	216	240

So here's how a pro bodybuilder—me—uses the same protein guidelines that you can adapt from the chart:

At competitions, I weigh 185 to 190 pounds. Let's say 190 is my ideal body weight. If I were not involved in sports whatsoever—didn't even jog—I would need protein by a factor of .5 grams times 190, or 95 grams of protein a day. If I were into jogging—or light fitness, training maybe once a week—I would need .6 grams of protein times 190 (114 grams of protein a day). Training three times a week, I would need .7 grams (133 grams total). Training daily with weights or aerobics on a moderate basis, I would need .8 grams (152 grams total). And if I was into heavy weight training every day, I would need .9 grams (171 total). In the last 12 weeks before a competition, doing a double split of exercises, I would need one full gram per pound of ideal body weight—or 190 grams of protein a day.

At 27 grams per average boneless, skinless chicken breast, and three grams per one large egg white, and 30 grams per typical broiled unbreaded fish filet, we're talking about a *lot* of chow. You might literally get tired of eating. In that case, to reach your quotas, you'll probably want to supplement your food with egg white powder or commercial amino acid powders. (As always, you shouldn't drink water from 15 minutes before a meal until 30–60 minutes afterward, or you'll have absorption problems.)

I carry a log with me and keep close track of those protein grams, and the times that I consume them.

If your protein intake matches your needs and your fat intake is low, you are doing exactly what is needed on the nutritional side to acquire tremendous muscle definition. The muscles you break down anaerobically come back bigger and stronger with the aid of your careful protein intake.

In the fall of 1991, I saw a tremendous difference in my own body from the Southeastern USA competition to the Mr. World. My body fat was four or five percent for the USA on October 5, and on November 23 it was 2.5 percent for the Mr. World. What I did was increase my protein intake from ¾ gram to one full gram per pound of ideal body weight. At the Mr. World I held more size, more "cut" and had less fat on my body.

Don't forget: This didn't happen because I guzzled protein. It happened because my protein intake matched my very heavy training load, and was spaced so that my body could use it.

14

So What's on the Menu?

I'm not in the cookbook business or the diet business. I wouldn't want to try to come up with a year's worth of recipes and peddle it as *Peter Nielsen's 365 Days to a New You*. That would be a waste of time. For one thing, only one reader in 100 would follow the regimen to its conclusion. That's why *Will of Iron* concentrates on motivation, on trying to show you so many good reasons for taking care of your body that you won't need a prescriptive cookbook under your arm in the kitchen and a personal trainer looking over your shoulder to make you exercise. For another thing, there's so much variety out there that a one-size-fits-all prescriptive diet won't work. Too much variety in people, too much variety in food.

Among people, there is first of all variety in taste. I grant you that if you are in the depths of a fat-laden, protein-heavy eating rut, you'll need to acquire some new tastes and modify some behavior. But you can eat healthy and still have plenty of elbow room for staking out your own preferences.

People also have enormous variety in exercise load. Now that you've seen some of what that means nutritionally, you know it wouldn't make sense to prescribe you a "diet" even if every reader was a 29-year-old male, 5-foot-10 and 180 pounds. If the heaviest weight you carry is a briefcase, and the farthest you run is to catch the Good Humor truck, then you need to look at a different menu than someone who is in a gym for an hour every day.

A third great difference among people is dietary abnormalities. That doesn't affect most people. But because of my lactose intolerance—and because of the nutritional counseling I do—I'm aware that the number of people with special problems is far greater than generally recognized. If you're lucky, it can be a blessing in some ways. I wouldn't have a pizza or an ice cream problem even without willpower; any dairy product makes me sick.

The variety in food—when you get into real food—is awesome. I mean, the difference between T-bone, New York strip and pot roast doesn't add up to much when you compare it to the zillion ways you can dress up a dish of pasta. Red meat is red meat and fat is fat. I can cook chicken breasts more ways than there are bars in Brooklyn. If you want, I can make them look like ravioli. Fresh vegetables come in and out of season, keeping you creative and keeping you from being bored. Once you realize what non-fat dairy products are all about, you'll be able to slop white stuff all over your baked potato without guilt.

So it really would be pointless and counter-productive to do the cookbook thing here. But after all this fact and philosophy about nutrition as it relates to exercise, it might be useful to give you a couple examples of healthy menus for two very different kinds of people. For good measure, I'll throw in a day's example of my own training diet.

A major key to success with any new nutritional regimen will be to put a little effort and creativity into tapping all that variety. There's an infinite number of ways to come up with menus that will offer the same nutrition. Remember what all these menus have in common is getting the fat out, getting the complex carbohydrates in, and fitting—and timing—protein consumption to match activity load. Those attributes are far more important than calorie-counting.

Goal-setting is a wonderful thing. And consciously thinking about what you put in your stomach should be one of your goals for the rest of your life.

The Couch Potato Family Plan

Here's four days' worth of a new eating regimen for your typical out-of-shape American who hasn't given much conscious thought, and no action, to a nutrition and fitness regimen. If you are overweight, you could actually use these menus exactly as written. More important, you can analyze the principles behind them and draw up your own.

Calories for each day add up to the 1,900 range. Unless you have a real obesity problem, I don't recommend any regimen that drops calorie intake to much less than 10 times your weight.

Chances are these menus show a drastic reduction in fat calories compared with what you're eating now. That's probably the single most important part of this plan. Carbos are high. Protein is from low-fat sources.

Remember to drink plenty of water through the day, but don't use it to wash down your food. In a perfect world, you'd bypass water with meals. If you're absolutely hung up on it, bring a small glass to the table and *sip*.

These menus deliberately plan for you to eat five times a day. Planning multiple mini-meals will help control your appetite, will see to it that when you eat you are eating good food, and will keep your metabolism rate higher. Be sure never to skip breakfast, and then to space each meal throughout the day.

Remember, if you are a serious couch potato with typical American eating habits, you will feel better and lose weight on this type of nutritional regimen—even if you don't launch a formal exercise program. Without exercise, however, you will *not* become fit. The beauty part is that if you eat this kind of food every day, your body will start leading you toward exercise. Nothing radical about that. Somebody with a 50-pound spare tire isn't real likely to hop off the couch and suggest a brisk walk down to the park and back.

DAY ONE:
BREAKFAST
3/4 cup (one ounce) of cereal
One cup skim milk
1/2 banana
Hot beverage

There's nothing like breakfast cereal to tune up your label-reading ability. What you don't want are fats (oils and nuts), sugar and sodium. Lots of cereals that tout high "enrichment" are loaded with all three. Plain old-fashioned oatmeal is a great choice. Plain shredded wheat cuts it, as do a few others—maybe five percent of the packaged brands on the shelves. The simple act of reading "breakfast food" ingredients can go a long way toward raising your nutritional consciousness.

"Hot beverage" is, of course, a euphemism for coffee. I've already preached my sermon on caffeine. If you're hooked, try to withdraw gradually. Cut back consumption. Give ginseng or herb tea a chance.

The cup of skim milk can be split between your cereal and your hot drink. If you've been drinking whole milk for 30 years, skim is going to taste empty. What you're missing is *fat*. Dairy fat is fat, just as sure as the stuff in your frying pan. After a few weeks of skim, you won't be able to stand the taste of whole milk. It'll taste like, well, *fat*.

SECOND BREAKFAST (2–3 hours later)
One bran muffin

LUNCH (2–3 hours later)
1/2 cup tuna, packed in water
One tablespoon fat-free mayonnaise
Two slices whole wheat bread
Lettuce, onion

Even today, store shelves are about equally filled with oil-packed and water-packed tuna. The latter gives you virtually fat-free calories of protein. The former takes the same thing and pours on the fat. More label-reading. More consciousness.

Notice the mayo is *not* "light," or "lite" or "reduced calorie." It's fat-free. Zero. Zilch.

Maybe you don't like onion. Maybe you do like tomato. Maybe you like dandelion greens! Whatever garnish you like from minimal-calorie fresh produce, pile it on.

"Whole wheat" means whole grain. Lots of factory-produced bread dodges the issue. "Wheat bread," for example. Of course it's wheat bread; we assume it's not made from zucchini. But is it whole grain? Seek out the real thing and after a week or two you won't be able to stand the puffy, fluffy, empty white stuff. Your digestive system will thank you.

AFTERNOON SNACK (2–3 hours later)
Small peach

See, this is the way diets read. "Small peach." Is it a *big* deal whether it's "small" or not? No. The big deal is that it's a peach, and not a chocolate bar or even a granola bar. Is it a big deal that it's a "peach." No. Don't buy a bushel of peaches. Buy a few peaches and a few apples and a few bananas and a few grapes—whatever. Variety is not only the spice of life, it's a cornerstone of good nutrition.

DINNER (2–3 hours later)
Four ounces chicken breast stir-fried with one teaspoonolive oil
    and 1/2 cup or more of mixed veggies: bellpeppers, broccoli,
    snow peas, mushrooms, onions,carrot slices.
One cup brown rice
Large salad with two tablespoons fat-free dressing, or flax oil
Baked apple

If you're not already into stir fry, you'll get there quickly. For one thing, it's delicious. For another, it's one of the easiest ways to be creative.

Scour the cookbooks for seasoning suggestions, then invent your own. Use a Teflon wok, or other synthetic-surfaced utensil, to get by with the least amount of oil.

Fat-free (as opposed to "light") dressings are now common in the markets. Again, scour the healthy cookbooks for homemade dressings that go light on oil or which eliminate it. Invent your own. Vinegar is a good starting point.

EVENING SNACK (2–3 hours later)

Small fruit

In fact, that stir fry, rice and salad might have been all you could handle at the dinner table. In which case, you still have the baked apple to eat.

DAY TWO:

BREAKFAST

Egg-white (two) omelette

$1/2$ cup fruit

You've got to be serious to get into separating eggs and tossing the yokes. But that is the one and only way to get out the cholesterol *and* fat. The frozen egg substitutes are indeed better than whole eggs if you can't handle it. But you know what? I've been eating egg whites only since I was a teenager, and they're delicious. Funny how food works that way. Habit. Habit. Habit.

To be specific, here's the difference between a whole large egg and an the egg white alone. Fat: six grams in the whole egg, 0 in the white. Cholesterol: 274 milligrams in whole egg, 0 in the white.

LUNCH (2–3 hours later)

Eight ounces non-fat yogurt

$1^1/4$ cups strawberries

Salad with one tablespoon fat-free dressing

Two whole wheat bread sticks

SEMI-MEAL (2–3 hours later)

One whole wheat pita stuffed with chopped veggies and sprouts, garnished with spicy mustard

      Maybe you'll want to cut it in half, for mid-morning and mid-afternoon.

DINNER (2–3 hours later)

Six-ounce flank steak

$1/2$ cup green beans

One cup cauliflower

One pat margarine

      The butcher shop used to keep the flank steak in the back room. It wasn't the thing you'd display with the traditional fatty cuts. Flank steak has moved out of the closet in a more nutrition-conscious era. Learn to cook it, and it's a good pacifier for somebody who grew up on beef twice a day. A couple of ounces are plenty, for example, to make a stir fry downright beefy. It is still beef, and it does contain fat—though much less than other cuts. Limit your six-ounce steak to a once-a-week treat.

EVENING SNACK (2–3 hours later)

Air-popped popcorn

      If you don't want to do the air-popper thing, microwave dishes are available that will do a reasonably good job of popping corn without oil. Which is, of course, the whole secret.

DAY THREE:

BREAKFAST

$1/2$ grapefruit

$1/2$ cup non-fat cottage cheese

Hot beverage with skim milk

SECOND BREAKFAST (2–3 hours later)
Oat bran muffin
1/2 cup applesauce

LUNCH (2–3 hours later)
Bowl of vegetable soup
Medium baked potato with 1/2 cup non-fat yogurt

If you get into cooking soups at home, you can control the fat content pretty easily—and make a delicious, storable meal while you're at it. If you eat soup from a can, buy the lowest-fat, lowest-sodium brand you can find. If you're in a restaurant, you're at the mercy of the chef. Obviously avoid creamy or cheesy soups. Don't be afraid to ask what's in the soup—or any other dish. There finally are enough health-conscious people around that any decent establishment knows by now it must be able to answer its customers' questions.

If you know you have a genuine low-fat or even non-fat bowl of vegetable soup in front of you, feel free to put a *light sprinkling* of grated parmesan on top.

Baked potatoes are a super example of viewing food through that second lens. Complex carbo. Healthy as all get-out. And, like most complex carbos, the only sin is in what you put on it.

DINNER (2–3 hours later)
Seafood primavera with four ounces scallops, four ounces shrimp, 1 1/2 cups fettucine, 1 1/2 cups veggies, sauteed in two teaspoons margarine

Primavera ordered off some menus, of course, would blow your dietary regimen out the window. If it's a good joint, they'll cook it this way for you (easily done) and save you from clogging your arteries with sauce.

By the way, let's pretend Day Three is TGIF (Thank God It's Friday) and very mellow. You might want to try a white wine spritzer with your meal. More soda than wine, and quite refreshing.

EVENING SNACK (2–3 hours later)
One small fruit

DAY FOUR:

BREAKFAST

$^1/_2$ cup oatmeal
$^1/_2$ cup skim milk
Two tablespoons raisins
Four ounces non-fat yogurt

LUNCH (2–3 hours later)

One bowl chicken broth
$^1/_2$ turkey sandwich made with whole wheat bread, garnished
with lettuce and veggies of choice
One small pear

SEMI-MEAL (2–3 hours later)

Other half of sandwich
One apple

DINNER (2–3 hours later)

Chili—made with three ounces ground turkey, $^2/_3$ cup red
beans, $^1/_2$ cup tomatoes, $^1/_2$ cup chopped onions andpeppers,
$^1/_3$ cup rice, $^1/_2$ cup salsa
Broccoli or other green vegetable as side dish

EVENING SNACK (2–3 hours later)

Frozen banana

A Regimen for the Rail

Most Americans would love to have this guy's weight problem.
But he or she represents a very substantial minority: people, mostly
teens and young adults, who are thin and frail, all skin and bones, and
need to put on some weight.

Just how bad is dietary fat? So bad that skinny people need to limit it. First, even thin people develop heart disease if their arteries are gunked up with cholesterol. Second, the idea is to add strong, lean tissue, not globs of fat. Adding muscle means exercise and complex carbos and protein—the same as it does for people of any body type.

The one day's menu plan shown below calls for a canned nutritional supplement. Many products are available from many manufacturers.

BREAKFAST

Eight egg whites
$1/2$ cup of oatmeal, cooked with water

MID-MORNING SNACK (2–3 hours later)

One 1,200-calorie gainer supplement (less than one gram of fat per serving, very high in carbohydrates)

LUNCH (2–3 hours later)

$1/2$ pound roast beef (lean) on whole wheat bread
One green salad with tomato
One tablespoon oil, plus vinegar (flax oil and apple cider vinegar would be my choice)
    A good alternate lunch would be two whole four-ounce chicken breasts and a pasta salad.

MID-AFTERNOON SNACK (2–3 hours later)

One protein shake: two tablespoons egg-white protein powder (25 grams of fat-free protein), one cup two percent milk, one tablespoon peanut butter, one banana and three ice cubes, all mixed in blender.

DINNER (2–3 hours later)

Two five-ounce pieces of broiled or roasted chicken or fish (whitefish, swordfish or tuna); or one 10-ounce steak
$1/2$ cup steamed broccoli
One baked potato or corn on the cob
Spinach salad

My Own Training Diet

This is typical of what I eat in, say, the last 12 weeks before a bodybuilding competition. For most of this period, I'm in the gym for about 2½ hours' intensive training every day. So anybody who thinks you need to load up on milkshakes and cheeseburgers to get the job done is obviously about 45 feet off-base.

BREAKFAST (5 a.m.)

10 egg whites

SECOND BREAKFAST (7:30 a.m.)

⅓ cup oatmeal, cooked in water, or: four rice cakes.

MID-MORNING SNACK (10:30 a.m.)

One broiled chicken breast and one frozen banana.

LUNCH (1 p.m.)

Two chicken breasts chopped up in a salad with one cup steamed green beans, one sliced tomato, alfalfa sprouts, one tablespoon flax oil, vinegar to taste, or: Two whole chicken breasts with a small pasta salad

MID-AFTERNOON SNACK (3 p.m.)

One protein shake with two tablespoons egg white protein powder, one cup apple juice and three ice cubes, mixed in a blender

DINNER (6 p.m.)

One six-ounce piece of broiled or roasted chicken or fish
½ cup steamed broccoli
One baked potato or corn on the cob
Spinach salad

I get "full." Honest. Food is habit, habit, habit. What you see here is plenty of nutrition to keep an *extremely* active human body fueled, to maintain weight, to replenish muscle that is broken down in exercise. Scientifically speaking, those are the only reasons we eat.

Do I ever "reward" myself with special treats. Yes, of course. But never while I'm in training. Out of training is another story, and it's this: My basic nutritional regimen remains essentially as simple and lacking in fats, sugars and salt as what you see above. I'll reward myself on a Friday or Saturday night, or on a special occasion, or on a vacation trip. But I never fool myself into thinking that a thick slice of apple pie, or a glass of Gran Marnier, is a part of my daily diet. The human body wasn't built to run on that stuff, any more than your car was built to run on kerosene. Fuel it wrong, and the repair bill might be so high that you have no choice but to junk it.

15

Nutrition and Kids (Adults, Listen Up)

The biggest tragedy in our whole dismal fitness picture is our kids. As bad off as the adult population may be, tomorrow's American adults look worse. You don't even need to see obesity. All you need to do is look at the stuff our kids are eating, and you can take a time machine snapshot 20 years into the future. It's not pretty. I don't think "tragedy" overstates the case at all.

One study says that obesity among children aged six to 11 has increased 54 percent in the last 20 years. Since obese kids are three times more likely to be obese adults, all those familiar remarks about "baby fat" are not only silly, they're lethal. Baby fat means there's a good chance you're getting an early glimpse of high blood pressure, high cholesterol and heart attack.

Those obese six- to 11-year-olds see about 10,000 TV commercials a year for food. *This* is the way we communicate in modern America. Ten thousand messages, and not one of them says any of the things I've talked about here. Seen any commercials lately for complex carbohydrates, packaged without sugar and salt? Seen any big-time jocks pulling down million-dollar endorsements to pitch bananas and whole grain bread? TV can be a marvelous medium. But mostly what it does to our kids is make them immobile, which is a crime, and train them to eat garbage, which makes TV a two-time felon. It's past time for parents, and any health-conscious adults, to get concerned about *this* kind of pornography, which has a well-documented effect on health.

A Harvard study projected that obesity among kids aged 12 to 17 increased by two percent for every weekly hour of television watched. A team at Stanford released a report recommending the obvious: a change in family lifestyle, including less TV time; more time together; more exercise—walking, cycling, hiking. Like the study suggests, you don't need a Nautilus or a health club membership to get exercise.

Many of our kids are getting into the yo-yo weight syndrome even before they're old enough for junior high. One study reported that nearly half of nine-year-olds and nearly 80 percent of 11-year-olds *had tried at least one fad diet!* Imagine: nine years old, already with a weight problem, already doing exactly the wrong thing to turn it around.

Health is more than the absence of disease. It is a whole life attitude. It includes physical and mental well-being. More and more adults have decided that it's *chic* to be healthy. They exercise aerobically. They eat low-fat diets. They drink less alcohol. The tobacco smoke is clearing (but is still present, tragically, among teens). But too many people are left out. It's still a minority of the adult population that has a grasp on fitness. Even those who learn to think fit seldom pass it on to their children.

Teens can learn a healthy lifestyle, too, just like the enlightened adult minority. Teens can dare to be different, can defy the microwave and fast-food culture. They can take responsibility for their own health, can even become leaders in their group. If you are a parent, you have a serious responsibility to do all you can to help your kids down that path. If you're a teen, you need to evaluate your own habits and think about where you want to be a few years down the line. If you're smart enough, for example, to know that education will put you where you want to be, then you ought to be smart enough to know that it won't be anyplace worth being unless your body comes along with you.

Most teens don't carry typical middle-aged bodyfat around with them. But teens especially need to understand that being fit is more than having a certain percentage of bodyfat, or being able to lift a certain amount of weight, or to run a certain distance. It involves an attitude of discipline and self-respect and self-love. A truly fit person is concerned with both body and mind. When your attitude is "fit," then everything else will follow. And your self-confidence will peak.

That's pretty preachy. Now let's get practical.

Nobody, let alone a teenager who is subject to all that peer pressure and all those hormones, can wake up one morning and say, "OK, now I'm going to eat right." Small, gradual changes are the way to go. Not only do they not turn your life upside down and leave you frustrated, but they are *lasting* changes. If you read the basic nutritional information in this book, for example—really read it, and understand it—then you can start to *think* about your relationship with the cheeseburger and french fries. I mean, are there *drugs* in those things? Does your social standing depend on you living on them? Use that second lens to look at your food. Do you want to open up your stomach and pour all that fat in, time after time after time? Some serious modification of your relationship with the cheeseburger and fries would be a small change in your life, but—nutritionally speaking—it would be an important one.

Don't try to live on spinach. But start making some substitutes: non-fat frozen yogurt for ice cream, non-fat yogurt instead of sour cream, a grilled chicken breast instead of a burger, a baked potato instead of fries, a bottle of sparkling water instead of a cola, a bagel instead of a bag of chips, a walk down to the park instead of spacing out in front of MTV.

If you're a teen, you should know that the experts say we adults can't reach you with that kind of message—it's too cerebral. You kids are living too much for today. You feel too immortal. Maybe so. Maybe that's the best way of explaining how fortunate I was to get a big-time message of mortality when Crohn's hit me at age 15. Maybe if it weren't for the Crohn's, I'd be in line at the pork shop right now. So you know I'm not blowing smoke when I say I was *fortunate* to get sick.

What happened to me at 15 was something that usually happens about 30 years later, in one way or another. Your middle-aged body sends you a message that says, "I'm hurting." Often it's too late.

That's why I want to keep trying, in every way possible, to reach kids—and their parents—with my message.

Nutrition is where it all starts.

Part Three

Sweat Equity

16

Starting at Ground Zero

A lot of words get tossed around loosely when people talk about physical condition. "Fit," for example. And "active." As in: "He leads an active lifestyle, and he's fit." Definitions of these words fall all over the map.

You know by now that my goal is to live to see an American society where most people are "fit"—particularly our kids, whose *un*fitness is a national scandal. Maybe your definition of "fit" is different than mine. For some, being fit means being able to get to and from the car without distress, or surviving last night's 10 martinis without an industrial-strength headache. I doubt if that's your definition, or you wouldn't be reading this book. For sure, my definition of "fit" asks for a whole lot more than that.

I think the *average* person should have muscle tone instead of seriously excess body fat; should have arteries that are not threatened by a junk-food, fast-food diet; should have enough cardiovascular endurance to change a tire or walk 20 blocks without feeling like he's in the ninth round of a heavyweight bout; should be free of the chronic debilitating effects of tobacco use and alcohol abuse; should be a person whose self-image—and reality—portrays a body in motion, not slumped on a couch with cooking oil on the fingers and TV in the eyes.

I think the *average* person deserves, and needs, the confidence and self-esteem that come with achieving these minimal goals.

And I think that if the average American resembled that version of "being fit," then an amazing number of us would be taking it even further, to the next step. That's because fitness is as addictive as alcohol or tobacco. Except that fitness improves and lengthens life, instead of deteriorating and shortening it.

Nutrition can win you just a piece of that picture. You also *need* exercise to be the best that you can be. Everything from your work day to your sex life to your ability to play a piano to your ability to *think* clearly is enhanced by the full fitness package. We're talking about improving the quality of life on so many levels that it boggles the mind. Any way you slice it, there's a very large empty space in the package if it doesn't include regular exercise.

The physical, mental and nutritional aspects of fitness are wrapped together so tightly that sometimes it's difficult to separate them. In this section, we're going to talk mainly about exercise; but let's back up a second and talk about this word "active." Here comes the mental part of the package again, because being active is really a state of mind, not of muscle.

You can't even begin an exercise program until you set the stage by taking control of your life in two ways: (1) getting your nutritional life into the reality zone, and (2) getting into an active state of mind. Step One we've talked about. Step Two means that you don't regard your body as a sack of bricks to move from chair to chair through the day, and then to throw on the couch until it falls asleep at night. Being active means the opposite of being passive, in what is probably the most passive society that ever existed. We are out of control, but not in the sense of a car barreling down a mountain road at 120 m.p.h. We're out of control in the sense of a car rusting in the backyard. We're sitting and waiting for the junkman.

And I've got news for you. When the body rusts, so does the mind. It's not just biceps and triceps that get put on hold when a couple hundred million human bodies vegetate in front of TV sets for hours on end. Whether you're watching *Batman* reruns or PBS, staring at the tube is *totally passive*. Even conversation stops. If you didn't have to blink and breathe, there'd be no signs of human life.

Maybe the best way to see this—like using that second lens on food—would be to climb behind your TV one evening and look back out the other way. Scary! Look at all those zombies!

I don't mean to say that TV is evil. In fact, I make part of my living from appearing on TV. There's nothing evil about chocolate, either. But we don't lie on our backs all night and let some high-tech gizmo dump candy down our throats. (At least I haven't heard of that one yet.) I'm just using TV as the common denominator of how incredibly *passive* Americans have become. The ultra couch potato sits and consumes pictures and chips and dip. He doesn't *do* anything.

Nobody knows how many black-belt couch potatoes exist in the U.S. today. But it's pretty obvious that a huge percentage of the population holds at least a brown belt in vegetating.

Sure, we work hard all day. The surveys say we're working more hours than we did a generation ago. But the surveys also say we don't have much energy left to do anything else. We're *tired*. Nine or 10 hours of crunching numbers or peddling widgets and we just want to plop down and recuperate. If you're a numbers cruncher or a widget peddler, don't take offense; but the human anatomy was designed to handle a lot more than that. The human mind might not have been designed to handle that much tension and stress, but that's a different story. Your passive lifestyle, in fact, has got you in a vicious cycle. Your mind has tricked your body into telling you it's too tired to exercise, when *just the opposite is true.* Eat right, get up off that couch, and—in a reasonably short period of time—you'll have more energy for peddling widgets and crunching numbers than you've had in years. All that tension and stress will be more manageable, too.

It's time to get into training. First the mind, *then* the body. You push the "active" button with a brain cell, not a muscle. The ultra couch potato—or even the brown belt—can't jump up and start playing a tough hour of three-on-three basketball every night, or running five miles every day. Those would be very decent ways of being active, but they would kill a couch potato. The ultra couch potato has nuked his or her body back to Ground Zero. He or she must very carefully, very deliberately take baby steps that progressively lead to increased physical activity.

It takes motivation to reverse years of bad habits and deterioration. That motivation has to come from within yourself. The main purpose of this book is motivational. But all any book, or speech, or personal training can do is light a spark. You have to keep the flame going yourself.

As far as I've been able to figure out in more than a decade of personal training, couch potatoes are people who don't really comprehend *why* they should become active. They don't really *believe* it'll make that much difference in their lives. "Sedentary" and "sedative" are dictionary cousins. Couch potatoes are too sedated by inactivity to focus on fitness. Many come to me for personal training only after a wakeup call in the form of a doctor's dire warning, or a divorce, or some other trauma. *That* kind of motivation most people understand. So, couch potatoes, listen up. Here is a wakeup call *before* the trauma. Here are some reasons for getting into a new, active state of mind. Trust me; they're real.

(1) Being active is a circuit breaker. It's a *vicious cycle* breaker. Physical activity eats up tension and frustration like a vacuum cleaner eats dirt. If everybody in the country took the active path all the way to fitness, the combined income of America's shrinks would drop 50 percent overnight.

(2) Physical activity does good things to your body that will make you live longer. That's statistically speaking, of course. Mr. and Mrs. Muscle could get hit by a bus tomorrow, just like anybody else. Purging your body of excess fat and strengthening your cardiovascular system can't guarantee that you won't get cancer or some other dread disease. But a fit body is far more likely to wind up on the positive side of the statistics. Studies prove that you can even dodge hereditary bullets if you are fit.

(3) You'll discover the meaning of quality time, and you'll have more of it.

(4) You won't be afraid to look in the mirror. This reason alone is enough to deprive the therapists of a fair amount of business. It's also the least important reason for starting down the active path. But I have to tell you that appearance is absolutely the single biggest reason that people show up in health clubs, or call on me for personal training. That's wrong, wrong, wrong. Looking good is a tremendous fringe benefit to exercise. It's great. Can't beat the feeling. But it

should be reason #4 for becoming active. If you don't get in tune with the other reasons, your whole exercise program—just like its motive—will be cosmetic, and it will fail. We'll talk a lot more about this later.

Those are four good reasons, by anybody's judgment, for becoming active. You can't buy the results, however, with anything but your own sweat equity.

If you are a true couch potato, the idea is *not* to put this book down right now, run out on the deck and start doing push-ups. Not unless you want, at best, to fail; or, at worst, to kill yourself. First, you must take those steps to do something about your nutrition. That will get your brain seriously engaged in the fitness process. Then you must take a close look at just how physically passive your whole attitude has become toward "getting through the day." And then you must change that negative attitude into something a whole lot more positive.

Chances are just about 100 percent that you're pretty disgusted with yourself, and ready for change. Otherwise, you wouldn't be reading these words. But running headlong into change will guarantee failure. Better to crawl. Persistently, consistently, a little farther every day. Start by taking stock of just how *un*active you are, and how you got that way.

Partly, you know, you are a victim of "progress." A century ago, "getting through the day" would have guaranteed that you would be fit, at least in terms of exercise. Things got done by hand and foot. Everything from washing yesterday's socks to getting down the road involved serious physical activity. People built and repaired things themselves. They planted and harvested gardens and farms without machinery. If they didn't walk, they had a horse, and they had to take care of it. Handling the reins for one trip into town and back was as much exercise as two years' worth of power steering. In case you ever wondered how so many people managed to live into and through adulthood without modern medicine, that's probably the best explanation. Getting through the day burned lots of calories and involved plenty of aerobic (and usually anaerobic) exercise.

Now compare that with your world, which you have come to take for granted. Do I even need to paint the picture? How about just one symbol for the whole high-tech thing: your TV set's *remote control*. What an active person does is to *take remote control out of his or her life*. That is, ironically, the first step toward really, truly being in control. You don't have to go back to the 19th Century. Just get back into your body.

When you go to the mall, don't blow your cool when you can't park the air-conditioned buggy within two steps of the store. In fact, seek a parking space farther out. If you're meeting a friend, take a brisk walk together before you start shopping. When you go to a store on Level B, bypass the escalator and walk up the stairs. Back home, if you're addicted to MTV, don't just stare at the thing—get up and dance. If you're going to a convenience store two blocks away, walk. If you're going to visit a friend 10 blocks away, ride a bike. Don't gripe because the kid hasn't gotten home to take out the garbage; do it yourself. Instead of watching some rerun, take care of a household chore you've been putting off. These are relatively painless steps, even for the most confirmed couch potato. Take them all, a few more each day.

In the process, you'll start to get your mind in tune with your body, just like you developed that second lens for looking at food. You'll start to remember that you *do* have a body, the one all those remote controls made you forget.

This is a wondrous, complex machine you live within—far more so than all the electronic toys that isolate your mind and muscles from the real world. You have about 600 muscles, in fact, and 100 million muscle fibers. Every movement you make—running two miles or blinking an eye or moving your food through the digestive tract—is done by muscles. In the couch potato state of mind, we forget all that. In the fit state of mind, we can never forget. It's the couch potato who performs some simple task and then the next day moans, "Man, I used some muscles I didn't even know I had."

That's not just a cliche. It's true for millions of Americans. They prefer to let their muscles remain anonymous. If they climb a tree for the first time in 20 years, or go on a hike while vacationing at the Grand Canyon, the anonymity disappears suddenly and painfully. If a couch potato gets a flat tire that takes him out of his 65 m.p.h. cocoon to do some manual repair for the first time in 10 years, he's liable to do a macho tire change and pop a bicep. These kinds of injuries—on the job or in day-to-day living—are enough reason to take fitness seriously. You can't assume that your body will continue moving, in its complex ways, as long as you live in it. When it starts creaking like a 120,000-mile car, you'll be trying to fix it a dollar short and a day late.

I believe the greatest secret in making this attitude shift is to make your mind work *for* you instead of against you. You do this by constantly thinking positive—even if what you're thinking about is negative, like 50 pounds of excess fat. And how do you do this? By setting goals. Goals are not ideals. Ideals are something way down the road. Maybe you'll get there someday. Goals are things you can attain today, tomorrow, next week, next month, this year. They are realistic. You can reach them and check them off your list, and that's why you'll succeed. Instead of failing, you'll meet one goal, and then set out for the next one. That's why it's not trivial and not silly to make walking farther from your car a goal when you go to the mall tomorrow. It's going to be a whole lot of days before you can check "minus 50 pounds" off your list of long-term goals.

Couch potatoes, believe me: Many readers who have advanced far, far past this chapter in their personal fitness regimen know exactly what we're talking about. They've been there. *Don't think you're alone.* You are suffering the national disease. You're no Davey Crockett blazing a new trail away from fatigue and low self-esteem. That's a positive in itself. You're not the first person dumb enough to let your body slide so far. Recognize that fact. Instead of letting your current condition be a negative dragging you even further down, take stock, set realistic goals, and move forward—knowing you have lots of company. You're not exactly coming out of the closet. Everybody close to you knows you're in there.

With a sound nutrition regimen and an active state of mind, it won't be long before you'll be seeking exercise goals a little more stiff than walking a few blocks to pick up the Sunday paper. If you're only a partial couch potato, you're already set for an introductory conditioning program. In either case, this is a good place to give you a warning/reminder: *Get a physical exam.*

Years of inactivity have put your body on course for a shock. A little soreness is nothing to worry about. A heart attack is. Before you start a program, get a checkup (which you're probably overdue for anyway) and tell your doctor what you're about to do. Ask him specifically if you have any abnormal limitations in exercising. While you're at it, tell him that you're on a low-fat, high-complex-carbo nutrition regimen, and that you intend to stay on it the rest of your life. His diagnosis for your whole plan probably will be: "It's about time."

17

Conditioning, Plain and Simple

Maybe it's just human nature. Maybe it's just the American way in the age of high tech. But so often when when we're tackling a problem, we do two things: (1) we run out and buy a gadget to do the job, and (2) we make it much more complicated than it has to be.

Take a look at a suburban two-car garage. What's in there, two cars? No. Gadgets. Here's a $500 snow shovel that'll scoop the white stuff up off the sidewalk and spit it on the lawn. Here's a $2,500 lawn mower you can ride on. Here's a $150 rake that *blows* leaves into a pile. Here's the invention of the century: a fishing line attached to an internal combustion engine (it whacks weeds). A lot of garages don't have room for any cars; they're too filled with gadgets. I shouldn't have to point out that every one of those gadgets is designed to keep your muscles anonymous. Household gadgets and being active usually aren't a good match.

So it goes when we decide to start exercising, to take those first small steps toward conditioning. Too many people think the only way to get the job done is to run out and buy a gadget. Some of these gadgets cost a *lot* of money. And most of them are complicated, even if they look like a piece of Scandinavian furniture. You have to make adjustments to do different exercises. While you fiddle around with the machine, you lose "the pump," that warm glow of a workout in progress that begs you to keep going *now*.

You *can* condition yourself on these in-home universal machines. But my experience has been that many people find them too intimidating; or, like a kitchen gadget that winds up rusting in the back of a drawer, people get bored with them. When somebody asks me about them, my usual response is something like: "You're probably better off to take your five grand, go back to the basics, spread the money over a couple of years and hire a trainer to come in and be your personal slave driver." I don't say that to drum up business, but because it's true.

Fitness is best approached plain and simple. That's especially important down at ground level, when you're not trying to win a Mr. Universe or a North American swimming title or a triathlon. All you want is to slim down, tone up and make your body start working for you instead of against you. You're trying to stay in an active state of mind, in touch with your body. The last thing you want to do is to go out and buy a high-tech gadget. Every corner of your brain associates gadgets with something being done *for* you. Fitness is 100 percent something you are going to do for yourself.

Make it simple. Make it fun.

Let me tell you, for example, about three plain and simple —and cheap—ways to give yourself a workout. The first one doesn't cost a dime. The second one uses a dime-store piece of equipment that probably is sitting in your basement or attic. The third one uses a piece of equipment you can buy at the drugstore for less than $5. All three are fun. All three can easily be done by recovering couch potatoes who have *never* worked out. But at least two of them are also practiced regularly by champion athletes. All can be done in the privacy of your own home—or in a motel room while on a sales trip or on vacation. These are workouts that remind me, in the best of ways, of when I was getting started back in my grandmother's basement in Brooklyn.

The first workout method is incredibly simple, despite its imposing name: *manual resistance training.* It sounds so formal, so heavy, so macho. But it's the least formal thing you ever heard of. As for macho, well, about all you need for equipment is a towel and a broomstick. No dumbbells, no barbells, no iron weights. I've done this on the TV talk shows. Here comes a guy (me) who looks like he's been training for years with megaweights, and he's running around the stage with a towel and a broomstick and another piece of equipment that I'll mention in a minute. Hey, anything to get people thinking fitness.

Before we even get to the towel and broomstick, you have to understand that there is a substitute for everything. Take two cans of tomato juice, for example, or whatever canned goods you have handy. Didn't know you had dumbbells on the shelf, did you? Start by walking rapidly in place, or jogging. Then pick up your "dumbbells," and hold them palms up with your arms straight down at your sides. Then, keeping your upper arms straight downward, raise one can up to your shoulder, then straight back down; while your left forearm is going down, use your right forearm to bring the other can up. You are now doing alternate dumbbell curls. First you did a little aerobics with your walking or jogging, then you did some resistance work with the cans. And you're starting to feel a nice burn.

You say you're too shy or embarrassed to go to the gym, at least not yet? Well, who's going to tell on you? The cat? He may be a little confused at all this activity, but he won't talk.

Anyway, courtesy of a couple of cans and your own creativity, you're now getting a little taste of "the pump." Take a 30- to 60-second rest, while shaking out your arms. Then use the cans again, this time in a lateral movement, with your arms starting at your sides and rising—together and slightly bent—to about ear height. Do 10 or 15 of these. Then take that 30- to 60-second rest, which is something you'll be doing between exercises even if you wind up pumping iron in the fanciest gym. Then do alternate front laterals—raising one arm at a time in a forward motion.

Now you're warmed up. We'll come right back to manual resistance training, but let's go for a minute to that other piece of equipment in your basement or attic. This is the one that I'm not aware of any champion athletes using, but believe me, it's one terrific form of exercise. We're talking *hula hoop*. This is one fad that never should have died.

Put on some music or MTV. Your cat is really going to laugh at this one, but who cares? Slip that old hoop over your head and start twisting. In case you forgot, the object is to keep the hoop above your waist. It's going to fall on the floor, guaranteed. Pick it up and twist harder. This is *very* tiring stuff. You are working your abdominals, your obliques, your intracostals, your back. If you are a true couch potato, tomorrow you're going to feel like you were hit by a sledgehammer—and you'll work it right back out. And if you're feeling silly at first, don't forget: *I* did this on TV and survived.

Seriously, the hula hoop is first-class exercise. In a small way, it's a version of the cross-training (aerobic and anaerobic) that we'll talk about later. Don't try to do the hula hoop all afternoon first time out. In fact, after taking a couple of minutes to remember how to keep the hoop up, twist your way vigorously through maybe just one song—about three minutes. You ought to be keeping a fitness diary, or log. Today you can write down something like: "Hoop: one song." Try two songs next time.

Now, back to manual resistance training—with a nice sweat worked up.

As with any kind of exercise, you'll get the best results if you have a training partner. So why not get your spouse, or a friend, or a parent—or a grandparent—involved? He or she can use the workout, and you can use the physical resistance and the moral support.

Take the bath towel and do some pulls. Remember that your partner's actions are a mirror image of your own. Whatever movements you make, whatever muscles you work, will be done on the opposite side of your partner's body.

Roll the towel up lengthwise, so it's like one long, thick rope. You grasp one end, your partner the other. Plant your left foot forward, with the left side of your body turned toward your partner, towel held firmly at stomach level, right hand in back and left hand forward. Your partner has reversed all that, and is planted on the other side of the towel. Like the name of the exercise says, you *pull*. Pull, breathe, relax, stretch while your partner pulls back; then repeat. Do the exercise to failure —when you start to feel a muscle burn; then reverse positions and do it again. You don't know what it means yet, but what you are doing is kind of a mini-version of supersets for your biceps and your back. Pull for biceps; stretch for back.

Now face each other and hold the towel horizontally. You grasp it, wide grip, palms under. Curl up. Meanwhile, your partner, palms above the towel with a narrow grip, pushes downward. Curl; breathe; relax. Do a vigorous set of 10. Take your 30- to 60-second rest, then reverse positions and repeat the exercise. Curling up, you're working your biceps; pushing down, you're working your triceps.

You see the concept. You can clone almost any gym exercise, as long as there's resistance. Weight training is resistance training, with iron supplying the resistance. Manual resistance is very light training, and you cannot build a Mr. Universe—or even a Mr. Saskatchewan—body by doing manual resistance. You *can*, however, burn calories and tone muscle. It is fitness plain and simple. In a way, manual resistance was made for the beginner. A 120-pound barbell will supply 120 pounds of resistance from now until doomsday. When a lifter tires, he's stuck. In manual resistance training, when you—or your partner—tires, there is less resistance.

You can tie a towel to a door or a heavy piece of furniture. If you've got a *long* towel, you can stand on one end. It's best, however, to have a partner. If you have a partner and a broomstick, you can even replicate some specific weight-training exercises. Still plain and simple. And fun.

You lie on the floor, for example, grasp the broomstick shoulder-width like a barbell and push upward—breathing out at the hardest part of the exercise. It's hard because your partner, standing above, is grasping the stick and providing downward resistance. Now you're doing benchpresses with no bench and no weights. All of the principles of weight resistance training—repetitions, breathing, rest, etc., which we'll talk about later—apply to these simple broomstick exercises. Remember, muscle starts to atrophy after *12 hours* of inactivity. You can't build masses of muscle doing manual resistance training, but if you have been inactive for, say, *12 years,* then you *will* build muscle with that broomstick, that hula hoop and that towel.

Now here's that third piece of equipment I mentioned. It's called the Dynaband. As you've seen, I'm not into touting specific brand names in this book, but this little jewel is something special. You can buy the Dynaband at most chain drugstores for less than $5.

They look something like a bicycle tire inner tube and they come in three different colors, for three different degrees of resistance.

Couch potatoes, kids, grandmothers and housewives can make good use of the Dynaband and have fun while they're at it. Pro bodybuilders use them to warm up backstage at competitions, or for a mini-workout when they can't get to a gym. I've got an old picture of Schwarzenegger and Sergio Olivia, a couple of champions, warming up together with Dynabands. I use the Dynaband myself, often.

Portable? Stick it in the corner of a briefcase and you've got a gym wherever you go. There's never an excuse for not working out.

Put it under your foot and do curls for your biceps. Do leg pulls for your outer thighs. Do arm pulls for your chest and shoulders. It's excellent manual resistance conditioning, as good as you can get without a partner. And, of course, you can do a Dynaband workout with a partner, too.

So what's the real point of talking about towels and broomsticks and drugstore equipment that looks like an inner tube? Creativity. Fun. Lack of intimidation. A door to the active path that's open to anyone. No matter how far out of shape they are. No matter how embarrassed they are. No matter how little money they have. No matter how little time they have. Once you become *active*—remember, it's a state of mind—you'll understand that exercise, and all its rewards, is right there for the taking. Instant gratification without spending big bucks.

The inactive person goes down to the lake on a Saturday afternoon and looks at the water. The active person—even if he can't swim from here to the dining room—discovers that it's incredible exercise to walk or jog in knee-deep water. It burns calories and is tremendous for the legs.

The inactive person watches America's Team on TV while a hired kid does the yard. The active person cuts the grass and whacks the weeds himself. He wears a hat, drinks plenty of fluids—and burns 550 calories an hour. He's in tune with his body, and he knows that he's doing more than using up an hour's time and making his neighbors happy.

I *love* the gym. Once you reach a certain plateau of fitness, there are things you can do in the gym that you can't do anywhere else. I work out on a half-million dollars worth of equipment, and it pays off. But I also work out with my Dynaband. And one of the best exercises I do, every morning at home, is half push-ups with my feet on the bed. Zero equipment, unless you count the bedroom rug.

A lot of this, of course, goes back to my grandmother's basement. And to Julie's gym, where champions were born but no awards were won for interior design. Plain and simple.

One day—maybe even right now—you might be ready for the gym. But it's not the only place to get exercise. And it doesn't have to cost a dime.

18

You Gotta Have Heart

Let's go back to that average out-of-shape driver whose air-conditioned cocoon blows a tire on the freeway. The suit coat comes off, the sleeves get rolled up, the jack comes out of the trunk. In a few minutes, our friend is going to get a double whammy. He is going to discover that he is seriously lacking in both kinds of fitness: endurance and strength.

Soon after lugging the spare out of the trunk and squatting down to yank on the lug wrench, he's sucking wind. Aerobically speaking, his cardiovascular *endurance* is about equal to the Happy 40th Birthday balloon that has been hanging around—barely—for a couple of weeks.

Then, trying to twist the fifth lug nut, he finds that right at the moment he probably couldn't twist the top off a pop bottle. His *strength*—something built up anaerobically through resistance against muscle, whether by weights pumped in the gym or by boxes unloaded from a truck—is non-existent.

There, in a graphic nutshell, you see some obvious reasons for conditioning your body along both fitness paths. Aerobics training and resistance training are two entirely different animals, but in the real world they go together like country and western. (Remember, we don't talk ham and eggs on our new dietary regimen.) Aerobics and anaerobics. Endurance and strength. Work on them both in a conditioning program and you can say that you're into "cross-train-ing." Imagine, for example, that you have worked yourself up to a three-day-a-week regimen—in your own basement—of 20 minutes of jump rope or hula hoop (aerobics), followed by a Dynaband routine (anaerobics). That would make you as solidly into cross-training as if you had a personal trainer and access to a million-dollar gym.

For starters, you need to know something about aerobics.

If you really are at a *starting* point, losing fat is undoubtedly one of your goals. Aerobic exercise is the fat-burning king. You could take your wife dancing and—assuming you stayed on your feet and the tempo stayed up—you could boogie off 600 calories in a very aerobic evening. An hour of working your way through a weight-lifting rou-tine—even if you power-lifted the Empire State Building—would burn off practically zilch.

The fat-burning qualities of aerobics is an attention-getter for couch potatoes (see Chapter 12). But the real reason for pursuing aerobic fitness is what it does for the heart. Aerobics, in fact, strength-ens the entire cardiovascular system. More oxygen gets to the cells that need it, and it becomes easier for your heart to get it there. An aerobically fit individual's heart beats about *17 million* fewer times in the course of a year. You don't need to be a physiologist to understand what that means.

In terms of performance, the big fringe benefit is endurance. We've got quite an endurance range in this crazy modern world where exercise is something we have to schedule into our lives. The air-sucking tire changer, for example, might be a salesman who works right across the desk from a marathoner. Both of them good guys, both of them kind to their wives and children, both of them wearing $1,000 suits, both of them driving big new cars. But one of them can run 26 miles and one of them can't change a tire. The wild thing is that I'm not exaggerating the comparison for effect. You'll find that exact Mutt and Jeff duo in the real world, in almost any office.

So what does Mutt have to do to get into some kind of cardiovas-cular reality zone, besides taking remote controls out of his life? Specifically, he should exercise aerobically three or four days a week, keeping his heart at its ideal target rate for at least 20 to 30 minutes. Here's what that's about.

Put two fingers on your wrist and take a pulse for 10 seconds. Multiply by six. That's your *resting heart rate.*

If you're a woman or an out-of-shape man, subtract your age from 220. (If you're a man in very fit condition, subtract half your age from 205). That's a calculation of your *maximum heart rate.*

To get your *ideal target rate* for aerobic exercise, calculate 60 to 70 percent of your maximum rate.

An aerobic exercise program means that you take your heart to its ideal target rate, sustain it there for a certain period of time, and do the workout a certain number of times per week. Different authorities suggest slightly different numbers for all those variables. The ones I follow are the American Heart Association (the ideal target rate of 60 to 70 percent of maximum) and the Institute for Aerobic Research (four times a week, 20 minutes per session; or three times a week, 30 minutes a session).

What's going on while you exercise aerobically? Your blood becomes more oxygen-rich, and at the same time removes more carbon dioxide from all your body's cells after delivering the oxygen. Your muscle cells become more efficient at processing oxygen and eliminating lactic acid (meaning you won't have the lactic acid soreness that follows anaerobic exercise). Your blood vessels become more flexible, so your heart is less taxed. Lung capacity increases. Your heart, itself a muscle, becomes better supplied with blood, and grows stronger. Your supply of HDL (good) cholesterol increases, while the supply of LDL (bad cholesterol) decreases.

And then there's your resting heart rate. An unconditioned person's heart may beat as much as 80 times a minute *at rest.* A person with good cardiovascular fitness will have a resting heart rate of 45 to 50 beats a minute. A superbly conditioned endurance athlete might have a resting rate in the range of 40 beats a minute.

Meanwhile, as we said when discussing nutrition, your basal metabolism rate stays higher even *after* aerobic exercise. So there you sit, burning calories and asking less of your heart. The beer commercials have it all wrong. It doesn't get any better than *this.*

If you work out too hard, you cross that anaerobic threshold. The heart loses all that efficiency in delivering oxygen and carting away carbon dioxide. You are no longer endurance training, and you will—in fact—have no endurance. You'll slow down, or quit, from exhaustion.

As your cardiovascular system becomes more fit, your anaerobic threshold will rise. More fit individuals can train at 75 to 80 percent of their maximum heart rate. Exceptionally fit individuals might even be able to train aerobically above 80 percent. Physiologists can determine your threshold with a treadmill test. The two-finger pulse check and the 60 to 70 percent target rate will work fine for starters. It's important to keep tab of your pulse, though, because you don't want to work yourself beyond the anaerobic threshold. It's not a health-threatening line if you cross it; but it will mean a quick end to the aerobic effect, and a quick end to your workout. (If you're chapter-skipping, by the way, we'll remind you that you should get a physical exam before launching any fitness regimen after a long period of inactivity.)

You can do specific aerobic exercises in the gym, or in your living room. But *any* exercise that takes your heart to its ideal target rate, sustains it, and doesn't cross the anaerobic threshold is aerobic exercise. A long, brisk walk in your Levi's, bringing your dog along for *his* exercise, is just as aerobic as running in place in designer tights while watching a $50 exercise tape. Jogging is one of the all-time great aerobic exercises. Many sports and activities, as we'll see in a minute, spill over—in varying degrees—to that gray area of cross-training.

Anaerobic exercise (literally "without oxygen") involves a quick, maximum thrust of energy. Aerobic exercise is a sustained, plodding activity in which the heart is stoking up the body with oxygen and burning up energy. Anaerobic exercise is a burst of effort that cannot possibly be sustained. Sprinting is anaerobic. Jogging is aerobic. Doing 10 bench presses with a heavy barbell is anaerobic. Flinging your empty hands into the air, *Dance Fever* style, while running in place is aerobic.

When you provide *resistance* against the sustained burst of effort, you are building muscle. Resistance is relative. Two hundred pounds of iron disks, for example, is stone cold resistance. The sets of exercises that make up a weightlifting routine are pure anaerobic resistance training. Don't tell a sprinter, however, that he is encountering no resistance when he drives off the starting blocks and pushes his body forward for 50 incredibly tense meters, trying to improve his time by a few hundredths of a second. His thighs will tell him there is resistance. (You could set a world dash record, by the way, without getting in a lick of aerobic exercise; at least not in the running of the race.)

A swimmer doing laps in relatively leisure fashion is getting a first-class aerobic workout. A swimmer dashing a lap is not exercising aerobically. He is, however, encountering real resistance from the water with every stroke. Put a pair of those floppy leather mitts on his hands and he'd be meeting resistance equal to a modest dumbbell.

Cross-country skiing is excellent aerobic exercise. Ask anybody who has tried it about the uphills, though. Plenty of resistance there.

So there is haphazard cross-training in most any recreational sport that involves sustained physical exertion and bursts of maximum effort. It is, however, just that: haphazard. And generally not very symmetrical. The thighs of a speed skater would be one good example. You generally can get aerobically fit by "going out to play." Anaerobic conditioning is more tricky. A full-body resistance training program is the only way to systematically strengthen muscles in all the body parts. For that matter, specific resistance exercises are the best way to strengthen any particular muscles that need extra work. That's why athletes from football, basketball, hockey—dozens of entirely different sports—head to the gym for conditioning.

An inactive person most definitely wants to get his or her conditioning program started with aerobics. Burn that fat. Strengthen that heart. Get that BMR raised. The benefits are all pretty obvious. Aerobics is the *core* of turning a flabby society into a fit society. It *will* tone muscle. Strength can be built in various individual and team sports. If the whole country were riding bicycles and rowing and playing soccer, I'd be deliriously happy. But it should be no great surprise to learn that I believe almost anyone can benefit from weight training, if they choose to try it. Most people would rather cut the grass, or clean out the cat's litter box. I think an amazing number would change their minds if they got into lifting.

What are the benefits?

First of all, if you're looking to build muscle, the weight room is the best place to be. No other game or sport that I know of directs work exactly to the muscles that need it, parcels out the work within a brief period of time, and puts you entirely in command of what happens to your body. We've come a long way just within my lifetime in terms of working a weight program into a total fitness concept. Instead of going into the gym and jerking macho poundage a few reps at a time, we warm up and cool down aerobically. The power-lifting branch of the sport still measures life by how many pounds they can put in the air, but most of us think in terms of overall strength, endurance and muscle tone.

Which leads us to the cosmetic fringe benefit. That applies to aerobics as well, of course, because cosmetic step one is to shed the fat. Cosmetic step two—the one that crosses the T's and dots the I's—is to replace the fat with some solid lean tissue. I keep saying this is the least important reason to be fit. But we do live in a *Vogue* and *GQ* world. The pressures to look our best are intense. Besides, firming up the old bod does wonders for mental health. It's a whole lot healthier and cheaper than plastic surgery. And it will give an excuse—a necessity—for buying some new clothes.

Back on a more important vein, don't let that buzzword "strength" get in the way of your thinking. "Strength" doesn't mean you're a musclehead. It takes strength to carry a briefcase and a sample kit to a dozen appointments a day. It takes strength to clean house. Our friend discovered it takes strength to change a tire. It takes strength *to get up out of a chair*. Strength is a part of everyday life for everybody. Your cardiovascular system *and* your muscles deteriorate every day you're inactive. Every *year* that you're inactive, the toll gets more serious. Until finally, a minor little unfamiliar movement pops a muscle or a tendon somewhere. Aches and pains often are a body's way of saying: "I've got no strength." Weight training is a good way to answer: "Here you are."

If you already are an active person, if you are an athlete, all the more reason to become a lifter. I've trained pro athletes from every kind of sport. All of them need specific strengths, and there's a way of improving performance in any sport through a specific weight program. A football linebacker basically needs to be able to push cattle around. A basketball player needs to protect and improve his already incredible leaping ability. Hockey players fly down the ice, but they need tremendous upper body strength to win those shoving matches in the corners. I trained a college quarterback known for his agility and flexibility. He was obviously not interested in bulking up with a heavy-duty anaerobic program. But he needed to keep his legs strong, and a program of supersets increased his endurance.

In other words, weight training—for all this talk about muscle— is meant to help you get to the point where you don't even have to *think* about your muscles. It's a way of getting ready for life's combat, whatever that might be: knocking down a lineman, changing a tire, cleaning a house, rehabilitating an injury. Weights—and other forms of resistance training—are a piece of overall fitness and well-being. Some bodybuilders become obsessed with it, for sure. But have you talked to any *golfers* lately? Or any Rotisserie baseball team owners? You tell me which is the healthier obsession: tapping a little white ball, reading last night's box scores, or building muscle?

The fact is, most fit people that I know in daily life away from the gym play racquetball or swim or play tennis. They walk a lot. What resistance training they do is with Dynabands and 10-pound dumbbells. They are at an advanced state of aerobic fitness, and that's where they want to be.

That's fine. Weights aren't for everyone.

But as you design a new lifetime nutrition and exercise path, kick a few tires. You don't buy a new car without checking out all the models and options, and your body is a lot more important than a new car. A health club isn't a bad place to start, even if you ultimately take your act back out on the road. A good club offers both aerobic and anaerobic options and has qualified staff to help you choose a path that works for you. A bad club will burn your money and waste your time.

If you can afford it, if you find the idea of going to a club to be a motivating factor for fitness, and if you want to test the various waters, here's a checklist of factors for choosing a club. Some of them may seem obvious; but I've seen every one of them turn out to be the difference between a good and bad choice.

- Is the club open when workouts will fit your schedule? If so, find out whether it has kept those hours long enough to suggest they won't change next month.

- Is it near your home or office? Ten miles might not seem like much in your initial enthusiasm. But what about two months from now when you're dragging after a hard day and it's time for your workout?
- What can you afford? Cost of membership varies widely. Some clubs have family plans at reduced rates. Many offer occasional specials for new members. If this is strictly a test drive, availability of a short-term membership might be a big factor.
- What about general upkeep? Are weight machines in good working order? Are the locker rooms clean? Take a good look around the place. If you don't want to be there today, you certainly won't want to be there in six weeks.
- How *well*-equipped is the club? Are there plenty of aerobics devices, such as walking tracks and bikes, and an aerobics dance floor? Is it a floating wood floor? Is there an adequate number of strength developing devices, including weight machines and free weights? Anywhere you have to wait for time with a device is a bad place to work out. You don't want to live there. You want to get in, have an intense training session, and get out.
- Is there at least one exercise physiologist on staff who is certified by the American College of Sports Medicine? It's important to have someone on hand who knows how to instruct you instead of just looking pretty.
- Are staff members certified in CPR? That's not meant to scare you. It's just another little sign that management is on its toes.
- Does it offer programs that interest you? Some clubs, for example, emphasize racquet sports. If you don't play racquet sports, you won't much care. The same applies to a swimming pool, which can account for a big piece of your membership fee.
- Are you looking for a place to meet friends, as well as to exercise? If so, does it offer a place for socializing?
- How much individual attention will you get? Is personal training offered? Will an exercise program be customized for your needs? Will it cost extra?

- Which items—massage, manicure, personal training, tanning, dining facilities, juice bar, etc.—are *a la carte,* and which come with the club?
- Do you know someone who is already a member? If so, ask him or her to rate the club. If you're lucky enough to have this option, it's one of the best barometers.
- Beware of gyms staffed by overly sculptured employees who are too busy staring at their own reflections in the mirror to help you find your way around. That isn't a physique; that's a musclehead.
- Visit several clubs and ask for a tour. Make all of your visits on a day and at a time when you would be likely to be working out. It'll give you a true sense of traffic. The same club that looks uncrowded at 10 a.m. might be a zoo at 5:30 p.m.—after work, and just when you'd normally be showing up.
- Don't join any club without first trying out the facilities. Many will let you do so free of charge, at least for one visit. If not, it's worth paying the one-time rate.

Some people have the discipline, and enough knowledge or self-study prowess, to get a genuine conditioning program up and running at home, on their own. Some people don't. If you fall in the latter group, *don't* be one of the thousands of people who don't try a club because they're embarrassed by their flabby bodies. This is where shopping around and kicking tires becomes vitally important. Clubs have diverse clienteles just like bars and restaurants. You don't, obviously, want to be in a power-lifters' gym. But you also don't want to be in a pleasant, attractive room where the emphasis is on socializing rather than fitness. Look and you'll find a place that meets a happy medium.

And, trust me, half the people in the place were wary, if not terrified, the first time they showed up for a workout. That feeling will disappear, along with the flab and the aches and pains.

19

What's in a Workout?

They don't call it a "routine" for nothing. An exercise program requires discipline of structure. Patterns in choosing the exercises themselves. Safety precautions. Warmup and cooldown. When you're doing the actual work, you're doing *repetitions,* or reps.

It all sounds so dreary. To be honest, on some days it *can* be dreary. Being fit doesn't mean you're emotionless, or that your biorhythms somehow hum into a single, glowing groove. One day you'll go into the gym or into the basement full of physical and mental energy. Another day, you'll be drained. It could be for a thousand reasons. You had an argument with your spouse or significant other; it was your birthday yesterday, and you made a serious departure from your nutrition regimen; you have a cold; your boss told you this morning that your paperwork was moving too slow; you're in the 10th week of a hurry-up, tight-deadline, 10-week project. Every day in your life is not the same.

Certain aspects of your fitness program, however, *are* the same, every time. Don't look at it as dreariness. Look at it as something dependable in an undependable world. Or as order amid chaos. Look at it as what a great musician, who performs to cheering crowds in concert halls around the world, does behind the scenes. Except that you've got it made compared to the great musician. Everything is turned around backwards in your favor. For every minute he's on stage, he has practiced scales for hours on end. For every week you're on stage, you spend just a few hours in the gym. You're practicing for *life*.

We're going to talk in this chapter about some of the basic elements and principles that make up a solid, safe, productive workout. We'll talk in terms of being in the gym, but you'll see that 90 percent of these pointers will apply if you're working out in your basement. We'll talk in terms of weight training, but you'll also see that 90 percent of what I say also applies to Dynabands and calisthenics and broomsticks and towels. These are the nuts and bolts of working out, and they are the same whether you are taking your first baby steps to fitness, or you've been pumping iron since the Korean War.

Partners

You can get fit, or sculpt your body to the best it can be, without ever once using a workout partner. But, man, is it easier—and safer—if you do the job two-by-two. I strongly recommend that everyone find a partner for his or her workout. A regular partner, of course, is the best.

Why is it best? For common-sense reasons.

Competition breeds success. This does *not* mean that when you enter the gym it's the bottom of the ninth, two out, bases loaded, down by three runs and you're the batter. It's not a *pressure* thing, it's a *motivational* thing. When that last set, or those ninth and 10th reps, require a little extra digging, it helps to have someone—even a friendly someone—on hand to see whether or not you do the work. (You're there for him or her, too, of course.) Don't forget that your partner is also in a me vs. me competition. He knows that it's not a question of whether you press 500 pounds, but how you stack up against yourself. When you make it through a routine with a 110-pound bar for the first time, you can *show off!* It works at every level—beginner or advanced. It's, "Look, Ma—no hands!" It's just plain psychological common sense.

Then there is what you might call the honesty factor. Not that I would accuse you of cheating. I certainly would never accuse anyone of cheating at golf, which is by reputation the most honorable of games. But how many strokes, on average, do you suppose we should add to all scorecards of golfers who play a round on their own?

Partners are a first-class safety factor. It's very much like swimming alone vs. having a "buddy." You get cramps, or hit a sudden wall of fatigue, and somebody's there to bail you out. In weight training, it's called "getting stuck." People have been seriously injured, or killed, when they got stuck with hundreds of pounds of iron raised above their neck. I really don't recommend anyone *ever* working with heavy weights unless they have a partner. And common sense suggests that anyone undertaking heavy exertion of any kind should at least have someone else in sight in case they become distressed in any way. (Safety should be a concern in *any* kind of exercise. Cyclists, for example, should wear a helmet. If you don't, try this one on for size: *Football players* are smart enough to wear helmets.)

Finally, it's more *fun* to work out with a partner. It's like the difference between shooting hoops by yourself, or having a little game of one-on-one.

Warmups and Cooldowns

A smart man doesn't hop into a $50,000 car on a cold February morning, start the engine and immediately see how quickly he can get from zero to 80 m.p.h. You don't do that to your body, either.

Warmups and cooldowns are a vital part of a routine, again whether you are doing towel pulls in your dining room or pumping 300 pounds on a lat machine at the gym. Even if your entire routine consists of two songs' worth of hula hoop, you should begin and end with a few minutes of running in place, holding your arms out from your sides and wriggling them to loosen them up.

Get your heart rate up and get more blood in the muscles. Get your breathing up to speed. In the gym before a workout, do three to five minutes of a nice, even, slow-to-medium pace on an aerobics device—a stationary bike, or a treadmill, or a stair machine.

Then do a few minutes of stretches. Muscles and tendons and ligaments can do an incredible amount of work. But do them a favor and help their elasticity ease into it. It'll help prevent snapping and tearing when you get to the heavier part of your routine. There are a zillion stretches and six dozen philosophies of stretching. A lot of it is idiosyncratic—meaning you find what's best for you. Make it a part of your self-education—from books and magazines, from personnel at your gym, from training partners, from self-experiment.

At the end of your workout, reverse the process. Do a couple minutes of stretches, then do three to five minutes of aerobic cooldown.

During your resistance-training workout itself, do a specific warmup for each exercise. In essence, do a super-light set (it doesn't count in your log or diary) that previews the movements for the muscle you are going to exercise. If it's a set of bench presses, for example, do a warmup set with just the bar, and no weights.

Breathing

Key organs of the human body have all kinds of backup capacity that most people don't use. Being your best sometimes means tapping into this reserve. We only use a minuscule part of our brainpower, for instance. And the average person only uses about a quarter of his lung capacity. When you're working out, you want to get as close to 100 percent as possible.

Breathing properly is a basic, essential key to any exercise routine. Your body needs oxygen, and it's not going to come from anywhere else. Your body needs energy, and the fuel you put in your stomach is only part of it. This is the other part.

Breathe deeply though your nose. "Deeply" doesn't mean jerking your shoulders upward to draw a big breath. It means breathing from the *bottom* of your lungs, from the diaphragm. Expand your chest as far as you can. (As you "learn to breathe," you're actually going to expand your rib cage and improve your posture.) While you're learning, you might even get a little light-headed—because you'll be high on oxygen.

There is an important rhythm to breathing while doing a routine. The best way to remember it is to *blow out on exertion* —in other words to exhale, strongly, during the hardest part of the movement. If you're doing bench presses, for example, blow out while you're raising the bar; inhale while bringing it back down. Practice the concept right now by doing some curling motions with your forearm. Force yourself to blow out while bringing your forearm up to your shoulder; exhale while lowering your arm. It might be just the opposite of your first inclination; but you'll feel the proper pattern, and get in tune with it, in just a couple of tries.

In the early days of your program, think about your breathing pattern constantly. Soon you'll be doing it right without thinking.

Remember, too, that proper breathing not only gets oxygen to your cells, it helps gets wastes carried away. If you don't breathe efficiently, you're going to be much more sore the next day. That's why all those huffing and puffing aerobic dancers avoid post-workout pain.

Body Parts

Being fit gets you in touch with your body. Designing a workout program gets you in touch with your muscles in an almost clinical, analytical way. There are six major muscle groups to be worked, and every exercise is aimed at one or two of them. More advanced exercises are aimed at specific parts of one muscle. In the routines I've designed, beginners work on all six major groupings in each session. As you become more advanced, and the work becomes more intense, that number decreases. For example, in my own training I work on two body parts per session.

The major groupings are chest, triceps, legs, back, shoulders, biceps. There are subgroupings, of course, such as calves and stomach. The object of a good beginner's program is to train—in a plain, simple, fun fashion—the entire body in a symmetrical way.

Study. Ask questions. Resistance training, in all its forms, has very specific goals for each movement. Know what it is that you are accomplishing, and you'll have more motivation to get it done.

Reps and Sets

This is where you keep score. Except the goal isn't to "beat" the prescribed number of reps and sets. It's to do them exactly as programmed. As you progress, the program changes.

The next chapter includes some of the workouts I've designed and used with considerable success over the years for everyone from beginners to advanced lifters. You'll see that the guts of each workout look incredibly simple: so many sets of a certain exercise, so many repetitions per set. But those numbers are very important. The number of repetitions in a set of a particular resistance exercise, in fact, determines what it is that you are doing to your body.

Here are the basic principles of reps—keeping in mind that more reps, of course, are done with less weight; and that larger muscles can handle, and need, more sets.

Is strength all you want? Do you want to bulk up? Then pure, unadulterated anaerobic exercise—quick, maximum bursts of effort— is the ticket. The power-lifters, the grunters for whom how many pounds they can hoist into the air is everything, look at eight reps as a *long* set.

Is definition and endurance your goal? You want to get your musculature "cut" or "ripped"? Then you're looking at basic sets of about 15 reps.

For me, 10 is a magic number. A set of 10 reps builds strength and builds muscle, but it also builds definition. In any basic program, think of sets made up of 10 reps each. Muscles that need more work get more sets.

Ten reps is a number *infinitely* more important than the number of pounds you are lifting. Gauge it this way, no matter what movement you are making: The eighth, ninth and 10th reps should be difficult. (To the point where an 11th might not be possible, or only with utmost effort.) When you are fitting that formula, the work you are doing is right for that muscle—whether the weight on the bar says 50 or 300. Ten *is* a magic number, and might be the most important thing to remember from this entire chapter.

Never sacrifice style for weight. If your biorhythms are down, or if maybe you haven't been able to get as much sleep as you should, remove some pounds from the bar if that's what it takes to get to 10. On the other hand, if you do 10 reps and put the bar down when you could be doing five more—then you should have added weight a long time ago.

Ten reps will break down muscle and stimulate growth of new, larger, stronger tissue. Remember to blow out on the toughest part of every movement, oxidizing the blood with each thrust of energy.

The number of sets is largely determined by the size of the muscle. The smaller the muscle, the quicker it will become over-trained. That's why a program might call for six sets of a shoulder exercise, and 12 or 15 sets for a leg exercise.

Don't forget that every single principle of reps and sets applies to manual resistance training—Dynabands and towels and broom-sticks. The magic number is still 10. And if you're a couch potato, you'll actually be getting enough resistance to build muscle.

Rest

Two different kinds of rest are vital to any workout program: rest between sets, and rest between workouts. Beginners need more of both.

Taking no more than 30 to 60 seconds between sets keeps you from losing "the pump," from losing oxygen-rich blood flow to the muscles you are working. Beginners will need all 60 seconds as a target rest period. If you're far enough out of shape, you'll not only be sucking wind, you'll hit your anaerobic threshold. You might experience some nausea, dizziness, headache, a cold sweat. If you lose your cookies, you won't be the first. Maybe not even the first of the day. It's all very normal. It's your body saying, "*Wait* a minute!"

You have to start out by getting your mind in tune with the fact that this is, say, a 40-minute workout; that it's a lot more than just the first exercise. Then you have to push your body, but not kill it. Let me try to put all this in perspective by telling you what typically happens with personal training clients who come straight from 30 years at the office to their first day in a conditioning program. What I try to do—what all good personal trainers do—is try to work them to the max, short of hitting that wall. They come in all rambunctious. They're paying me by the hour. They want to get it on. But I fake them out a little, give them as much confidence as possible, keep them from feeling intimidated—but only give them *half* the workout. Next time, they get more.

Get the picture? *You* are the sculptor in every step of this conditioning process. You will constantly get in greater touch with your body. In the first workout or two, it might be more like your body slapping you in the face. You have to have patience with your body, listen to it, push it but don't insult it. You have to *wean* into fitness. You want to be back in the gym again and again for the rest of your life. Don't intimidate your body into refusing to bring you back.

I do "instinctive training." If I'm supposed to be doing five sets of one particular exercise, and if I lose "the pump" after four sets, I drop it. I move on. I've reached the plateau for that exercise. It takes *years* to be that in tune with your body. It's worth it in so many ways. Like when peer pressure or convenience tells you to pick up a double cheeseburger. A fit body tells you many things you can't hear just yet.

Rest between workouts is also crucial. A beginner will need 24 to 36 hours to recuperate. It takes me 12 hours—but again, it took me years to get to that point. Most beginners I put on a three-day-a-week program, two exercises per body part, two to three sets per exercise, 10 reps per set, 30 to 60 seconds between sets. That will build a foundation. There will be soreness in the first few rest days, but it will quickly diminish as you continue to work out.

Supersets, Tri Sets, Giant Sets

These exercises have a kind of Superman sound to them, but they are really just the opposite of power-lifting. They add aerobics and endurance conditioning to resistance training. They are very effective for athletes in endurance sports, who also want to add to their strength. I used supersetting, for example, to help condition a pro basketball player who was coming back from an achilles tendon injury.

Supersets are nothing more than two different exercises, one set each, done back to back without rest. I use supersets myself for aerobic conditioning. And in the final weeks before a bodybuilding competition I use tri sets (three exercises back to back with no rest) and giant sets (four or more) to add tremendous definition to the musculature I have built in months of workouts.

The intensity in supersetting is immense, but there's no reason to be wary. The most effective supersetting is done on the *same* body part—chest, for example—in two different exercises. You'll be dissecting the muscle, exercising it in separate places, using its reserve energy and bringing it to maximum exhaustion. That's the key.

Any workout should aim to get in and out of the gym quickly —building muscle without overtraining, or getting stale, or getting bored. Neither you nor your muscle will get bored with supersets. In fact, you'll "confuse" the muscle and fake out its "memory"—the reason your body becomes immune to a single exercise routine if you follow it too long.

A superset shocks the body, throws it a curveball. Doing two different exercises back to back with *no rest* moves the intensity from second gear to fifth gear. You'll be cross-training, doing aerobics and anaerobics simultaneously.

You use less weight and, once again, the magic number of 10. When you complete one superset, you take the usual rest period (30 to 40 seconds, because you'll be conditioned before you do supersets). That's a fast pace, and you'll probably be sucking wind. Your cardiovascular endurance will thank you for it.

Bodybuilders aren't building muscle with supersets and lighter weights, they're sculpturing—which is why it's a pre-contest routine. As a combined endurance/strength workout, it's dynamite for a triathlete, a downhill skier, a tennis player or a basketball player.

Because of supersetting's aerobics component, it's also the perfect exercise for someone who wants resistance training but also wants to lose some weight. A high-carbo, medium-protein, low-fat nutrition regimen and a gym regimen of supersets will make him or her one lean person.

Safety

Gyms can be dangerous places. So can cars. Defensive drivers who wear their seat belts shouldn't be afraid to drive to the grocery store. So it goes with gym training.

Some basic points:

Make sure you are constantly bending your knees while doing

any standing exercises. Your knees will act as a shock absorber. Otherwise your back will take the weight like throwing cement into a truck with no springs.

Don't lock out on certain movements. For example, military shoulder presses, squats, leg presses.

Wear a belt that's four inches wide. It'll also help protect your back. Anything wider than four inches will limit your range of motion.

If you don't want calluses, wear a snug pair of gloves. If you wish, use a little chalk for a better grip.

Wear loose clothing. You want good circulation and ventilation. Your arm can expand as much as an inch or inch and a half in the course of a workout, by the way.

Wear sneakers or running shoes, with the laces well-tied. You want support; and you don't want to trip.

Wear gym socks to absorb sweat so you don't get bacterial infection.

Always use a collar on a bar or adjustable dumbbell and fasten it tight to keep weights secure. That seems simple enough, but I've seen careless people splatter their face with a dumbbell.

When you're walking around a gym don't lean against equipment unless you very consciously know exactly what the equipment is and what you are doing. Gym equipment has moveable parts. Some are chain-driven, for example. You could leave a finger in there if someone decided to lift while your hand was in the way.

Keep a towel to wipe off your own sweat, or somebody else's, from a device or a bar you are about to grip or a bench you are about to lie on.

Don't work beyond your comfort zone in hot and humid weather.

Remember, "no pain no gain"—if you follow it out the window—is a fallacy. If something is painful while you're exercising, slow down or stop until the pain subsides. Overuse of muscles can cause damage or make you abandon your program.

Diary

Whether it's a 49-cent spiral notebook or an executive logbook, this is one powerful tool. To my mind, it's absolutely essential for a successful program. You *are* going to make progress. But without a diary, you'll be at times like a ship passenger looking out at the ocean to see how far you've gone.

Use the diary to keep an accurate record of when you work out, what exercises you do, how many sets and reps, what poundage you use. Keep notes of what seems to be working and what doesn't. At the end of a session, if you think you're ready to make a change in a particular exercise next time, note it down so that you do. Write down questions you want to ask a trainer or instructor who isn't handy at the moment.

You might find it useful to combine a nutritional diary with your exercise diary. You should be keeping both. Some people find it easiest to put them in the same place; some find it more difficult.

Progress is all about goal-setting. After you've worked out a few months, and you hit a psychological down point (we all do), almost nothing will help you out as much as looking in your log. You'll see where you were. You'll remember why you're doing this. And you'll understand that, yes, you're getting there.

Fluids and Fuel

Drinking fluids before, during and after a workout is important. So is the timing of your food intake. Be sure to refer back to Chapter 12 for details.

20

Five Levels, Five Programs

Every body is different. Whether you are training at your home alone, at a gym with a partner, or with a personal trainer, you'll find ways of customizing any exercise regimen to your needs. In fact, you'll be changing your routine from time to time just to fight off that old enemy, boredom. So it's impossible to line up a set of exercises on the pages of a book and say, "Here; this is what you should do."

What we *can* do is take a look at five very different programs for five very different people. If you fit the profile of any of these people, you could pick up the routine and use it just as it's written. Very soon, however, you would begin to alter the routine, gradually, to match your progress, your current interests, any upcoming competitions or lifestyle changes, etc. Creativity in the gym is just as important as creativity in your nutritional regimen. You don't want to go stale, and get off track.

Manual Resistance Routine

Remember, manual resistance is a great exercise tool for anyone: from couch potato to football player to bodybuilder. This routine makes use of three pieces of equipment—a bath towel, a broomstick and a Dynaband. Keep in mind that Dynabands come in three different resistance strengths to match your physical condition.

This routine works out all the basic body parts, and is perfect for a beginner—who should seriously consider working out with a partner, both for motivation and for fun. More advanced conditioners should never scoff at manual resistance training. It'll help keep you toned, and it means you never have an excuse for missing a workout, no matter where you are. Remember, an experienced gym rat can replicate almost any weight resistance exercise with a manual resistance equivalent.

CHEST Three sets of 10 reps	**EXERCISE** Flat flyes done on bench or floor, with Dynaband or with hand resistance

Lie back on the floor or on a bench, holding the Dynaband in each hand above the chest with a palms-in grip. Slowly lower Dynaband out and down until arms are parallel to the floor, maintaining a slight bend in the elbows. When pectorals are fully stretched, change direction and raise back up while tightening the chest muscles. Always take a deep breath as you move downward; blow out and constrict the muscle as you move up. That's one rep. (Without a Dynaband, have your partner provide hand resistance to both downward and upward movements.)

SHOULDERS Three sets of 10 reps	**EXERCISE** Seated military shoulder press, behind neck with broomstick (requires partner for resistance)

Sit down against back of chair to keep back straight and to provide support. Grasp broomstick with hands slightly beyond shoulder width. Begin with stick behind head and almost touching vertebra at base of neck. Push up. As you're thrusting up and blowing out, your partner provides resistance. When you get the broomstick three-quarters of the way to full extension, start bringing it back down. (Do not lock out elbows, or you could injure yourself.) Your partner, of course, must provide resistance in both upward and downward movements.

BACK	**EXERCISE**
Three sets of 10 reps	Towel pulls
BICEPS	**EXERCISE**
Three sets of 10 reps	Bicep curls, with towel or broom-stick or Dynaband

---

For curls, stand upright, or sit, holding broomstick, towel or Dynaband in a shoulder-width grip with palms up. Your partner will have a close grip, palms down. Raise hands while keeping elbows locked to your sides so the only part of the arm you're using is from hand to elbow, with the elbow serving as pivot. Constrict the biceps as you raise broomstick or Dynaband or towel almost under your chin. Lower arm nice and slow—all the way until device touches thigh. That's one rep. Blow out coming up, the toughest part of the motion.

| **TRICEPS** | **EXERCISE** |
| Three sets of 10 reps | Tricep pushdown, with towel or broomstick or Dynaband |

Instead of palms facing you, as in curls, place your hands—and thumbs—*over* the towel or stick or Dynaband. Use a close grip, with your hands touching each other. Your partner uses a wide grip, outside your hands. (As you do triceps, he or she does biceps.) Keep your elbows tucked into your sides, as if a pin went through your body to keep them in place. As you move downward you do want to lock out, to squeeze and constrict the tricep. Do not take elbows away from sides as you come up.

LEGS	**EXERCISE**
Three sets of 10 reps	Side leg lifts, with Dynaband or hand resistance; leg extensions, with towel or hand resistance

For leg lifts, lie on side with Dynaband totally encircling both ankles. (Without a Dynaband, have partner supply resistance.) Lift leg in a "splits"-type movement, then turn on other side and repeat set with other leg. This is great for hips and buttocks.

To build the quadriceps (front of thighs), do leg extensions. Sit down on chair with resistance of hand or someone holding a towel over your ankles. Keeping the back part of your knee touching the end part of the chair, bring legs up together with toes pointed upward. Squeeze the quadricep. And do lock out at the top, hesitating for a second while squeezing the muscle.

HAMSTRINGS	**EXERCISE**
Three sets of 10 reps	Resistance with hands, towel or Dynaband

Lying on your stomach, you move against resistance to the back part of the ankle as you raise the lower legs upward, using the knee as pivot point. Raise both legs together, from knee to ankle. Then move back down—again against resistance. This exercise strengthens lower back as well as hamstrings.

Beginner's Weight Program

This is one I designed for a corporate fitness program, but it's basically adaptable for any beginner. Remember, it's not about the amount of weight; it's about the reps and the magic number 10. Do *not* injure yourself by starting out with too much poundage. You can always add more until the ninth and 10 reps are difficult. That will be your benchmark for the time being.

All my beginner's programs are designed for three days a week, Monday-Wednesday-Friday or Tuesday-Thursday-Saturday. Those two days off at the end of the cycle aren't just for scheduling convenience. They represent a proper cycle of rest.

This program is suitable for anyone who has never picked up a weight, or has been away from resistance training for a year or more. It will build a great foundation for moving on to the next plateau.

Warm up for five minutes on a stationary bike. Cool down after workout for five minutes on the stairs or a stair machine.

CHEST	EXERCISE
A: Two sets of 10 reps	A: Inclined bench press with barbell
B: Two sets of 10 reps	B: Flat dumbbell flye

For the bench press, use a 45-degree incline. Lie back and hold a weighted barbell above the chest at arm's length, gripping a little beyond shoulder width. Slowly lower the bar to the chest by bending the elbows. Lightly touch the bar against the upper chest, then press back upward until arms are straight. Pause and repeat. Blow out on exertion, going up.

For the flye, lie back on flat bench holding a dumbbell in each hand above the chest with a palms-in grip. Slowly lower the weights out and down until the arms are parallel to the floor, maintaining a slight bend in the arms to avoid hurting arms or shoulders. When the pectorals are fully stretched, change direction and raise the weights back up, tightening your chest muscles.

BACK	EXERCISE
A: Two sets of 10 reps	A: Wide-grip barbell bent-over rows
B: Two sets of 10 reps	B: Lat machine pulldown behind neck

For the bent-over rows, stand on the floor—or on a raised platform to get more of a stretch. Bend forward, keeping knees slightly bent. (This will serve as a shock absorber.) Grasp weighted barbell with wide overhand grip and lift bar slightly while your back is parallel to the floor. Keeping the back flat, exhale and bend arms to lift the bar until it is near the stomach. Inhale as you lower bar to starting position without letting the weight touch the floor. That's one rep.

For the pulldowns, sit at a lat pulldown machine gripping the long bar with a wide, open-handed grip. Place your thighs under the pads to hold the body down as you pull. Begin with arms straight over your head. Pull down by bending the elbows and squeezing the lat, stopping when the bar touches the back of the neck. Stretch the arms back out and repeat.

TRICEPS	EXERCISE
A: Two sets of 10 reps	A: Dumbbell kickbacks
B: Two sets of 10 reps	B: Tricep dips

For the kickbacks, grasp a dumbbell you can handle easily with one arm. Assume a bent-over position on a bench or stool or chair. Place one foot 12 inches in front of the other, with your upper body parallel to the floor. Hold the dumbbell with an overhand grip—taking care to keep your upper body and elbow in line, with your forearm hanging straight down. That's the position. The movement: While keeping your body still and upper arm tucked into your side, exhale and extend the arm (the only part of the arm that's moving is from elbow to wrist) to the rear until the arm is straight back. Inhale and return the dumbbell to the bottom position. After doing 10 reps, switch arms. This one will work the entire triceps.

For the dips, place two benches parallel and three to four feet apart. Support yourself on both benches—legs straight out and feet on one bench, hands behind hips on the other bench. Keeping the upper body erect, bend the elbows and lower your buttocks down near the floor. Use triceps to push back to straight arm position. Inhale moving down; exhale moving up. Squeeze triceps at the top. For added resistance you can place a weighted dumbbell or a plate on your thighs. This is a simple exercise you can do at home using chairs or a bed. The closer your arms are behind you, the harder the effort on your tricep.

BICEPS	EXERCISE
A: Two sets of 10 reps	A: Standing barbell curls (medium grip)
B: Two sets of 10 reps	B: Alternate dumbbell curls, seated

For the barbell curls, stand with feet at shoulder width, gripping bar at thigh level—with elbows nearly straight, palms facing upward and hands just outside the hips. Keeping the back straight, exhale and curl bar up to chest by bending elbows. Stop when biceps come fully tight, and do *not* let them relax by resting the bar against your chest. Lower bar while inhaling. This simple, classic exercise is great for bulding big biceps.

For the alternate dumbbell curls, sit upright on a bench or chair holding a dumbbell in each hand with a palms-in grip. Keeping the right hand immobile, twist the left hand so palm faces you and lift the dumbbell by bending the elbow. Squeeze at the top so you are flexing the muscle. Pause and lower to original position. Repeat with opposite arm, and continue to alternate.

SHOULDERS	EXERCISE
A: Two sets of 10 reps	A: Seated military shoulder press
B: Two sets of 10 reps	B: Dumbbell side lateral

For the press, sit on a flat bench with barbell resting on shoulders and gripping bar beyond shoulder width with palms facing forward. Keep back straight and feet planted firmly on the floor. Exhale as you press the bar to arms' length in a controlled manner. Inhale and slowly retrun the bar to starting position.

For the lateral, stand with legs spread wide, knees slightly bent and back upright. Hold a dumbbell in each hand with palms facing the body. Breathing through your nose, inhale as you slowly raise dumbbells up and out to the sides, stopping when arms are at ear height. Hold for a count of three seconds, then slowly lower weights back to starting position. Keep thumbs pointed upward at all times. Beginners may lift to a point parallel to floor and try to go higher as they become stronger. In any case, never lift above your head in this exercise.

LEGS	EXERCISE
A: Two sets of 10 reps	A: Leg extensions
B: Two sets of 10 reps	B: Leg curls

Extensions will build the outer front thigh, the quadricep. Sit at a leg extension machine with your insteps behind the roller pads and your hands gripping handles at the side of machine. Slowly straighten legs to lift the weights, keeping toes pointed up. Stop when knees are locked and quadriceps are flexed. Pause and lower, under control, to starting position without letting the weights come to rest. This exercise increases overall knee strength, boosts vertical jump and helps running speed. Be sure to adjust the leg extension seat so the back of the knee is snug against the front edge of seat. The bottom pad should be just above the ankle area but below the shin.

Keeping your toes standing at attention makes sure that you work the entire quadricep. Use a fluid, slow motion.

For the second exercise, lie on a leg hamstring curl machine with your heels beneath the roller pad and your chest flat on the bench pad, holding onto handles for support. Exhale and bend knees to lift pad as far as possible. Hold the flex position momentarily before inhaling and lowering to starting position. The kneecap should be just off the pad, or you'll hurt your kness. Keeping the heel tucked in isolates the muscle you're working. Make sure that it's a fully controlled, fluid motion.

STOMACH	NIELSEN'S TRI SET
Two giant sets, all to failure	A: Leg raises on stand
	B: Crunches (legs on bench)
	C: Sit-ups on board

Unlike all other muscles, the stomach area should be worked to failure instead of counting reps and resting between sets. As soon as you reach failure on one exercise, you move on to the next.

First, do leg raises on a legstand and work the stomach from the belly button down, attacking that little pouch area that a lot of people want to tone up. Because they work the lower abs best, knee tuck leg raises should be done first in routine. Position yourself on a standing abdominal chair, supporting body weight on the forearms and hanging the straightened legs downward. Keeping your knees nearly straight, exhale and bend at the hips, lifting the legs out and up in front of you until they are parallel to the floor. Pause and inhale while returning to starting position. Immediately repeat, using a slow motion to work the abs better and ease strain off the lower back.

Next do crunches with your legs on a bench and your back firmly on the floor so your body lies in three nearly straight lines—torso on the floor, hips to knees straight upward, knees to feet on the bench and parallel to the floor. Position your butt very near the bench (or the bed or couch; this is an exercise you can easily do at home). Make fists and cross your hands on your chest to centralize your weight.

Your arms weigh at least three to five pounds, and you don't want to put them behind your head as in a traditional situp. To start, push your neck forward, then—from the middle of your back to the shoulders—raise your upper torso three to four inches and *squeeze* (simultaneously blowing out). That's the crunch: kind of like half a situp, squeezing the muscles together. It's great for the stomach muscles from the belly button up. It's also "patient friendly" for people who have back problems.

For the situps, never use a board slanted more than 45 degrees. This exercise works the entire stomach, but again focuses from the belly button upward. Again, centralize your weight by crossing your fists over your chest. Sitting on a slanted board, go down just halfway, inhaling. Blow out as you come up fully and extend your neck so you're actually squeezing stomach muscles. As you blow out, you constrict stomach muscles and put tension from your own weight on your abdominals. Do this to failure—till you get that burn in your stomach.

CALVES	EXERCISE
Three sets of 10	Seated calf raises

Sit on a calf-raising machine with your knees under the pads and the balls of your feet on the front platform. Lift weights by raising the toes. Unlock the holding bar. Begin with heels lowered so that the calves are stretched. Exhale and lift the weight by flexing the calves and lifting heels as high as possible. Squeeze momentarily, then lower to stretch position while inhaling. Do three sets: first with feet straight, second with toes and feet facing inward, third with feet facing outward. This develops the full calf muscle.

Intermediate Weight Program

A person undertaking this program probably has been involved in weight training for at least a year. He or she already has built enough endurance to train four days a week instead of three—and will be familiar with most exercise terminology. (In any case, I won't define or explain movements we've already discussed).

By going to a four-day-a-week program, he or she is taking a serious step. Following this routine will allow you to be the sculptor, to customize your body—for size, strength, toning, speed, or for competition in any sport.

The program is designed for rest days on Wednesday, Saturday and Sunday. Day One of the routine (chest, triceps and legs) is done on Monday and Thursday. Day Two (back, shoulders and biceps) is done on Tuesday and Friday.

Stretch and do at least five minutes on stairs, bike or treadmill for warmup.

DAY ONE

CHEST:	A: Incline bench press with barbell	5 sets, 10 reps
	B: Incline dumbbell flyes	3 sets, 10 reps
	C: Flat bench press with barbell	5 sets, 10 reps
	D: Flat dumbbell flyes	3 sets, 10 reps

TRICEPS:	A: Over-the-head one-arm dumbbell tricep extensions	2 sets, 10 reps
	B: French press, lying down or on bench with close grip	3 sets, 10 reps
	C: Pushdowns on lat machine	3 sets, 10 reps

For the one-arm dumbbell tricep extensions, stand upright with your left hand on hip while holding a dumbbell above the head in the right hand. Begin with upper arm tucked into the ear, elbow bent so the weight is behind the head. Without moving the upper arm, exhale; then straighten the elbow until the weight is above you and triceps is flexed. Inhale while lowering back down behnd the head, bending the arm only from the elbow to the wrist and extending the triceps. Your biceps remains tucked into the side of your head. Complete a set, then alternate with the other arm.

For the French press, lie down on a flat bench and grasp the barbell with a close grip, palms away from your body. Take the bar off the rack and hold it over your chest with arms fully extended. Your elbows are going to stay stationary and tucked, while your forearms lower the bar to forehead level. Inhale as you are coming down, blow out and extend the triceps as you go back up. In truth, this is a tough movement—and excellent triceps developer—in both downward and upward motions.

LEGS:	A: Squats	5 sets, 10 reps
	B: Leg extensions	4 sets, 10 reps
	C: Leg press	5 sets, 10 reps
	D: Leg curls	4 sets, 10 reps

For squats, hold the weighted barbell on your shoulders and assume a shoulder-width stance. Standing with your heels on a two-by-four will provide better leverage and put more emphasis on the quadriceps. Hold the bar beyond shoulder width, with palms over the bar, and keep the head up and back straight. inhale deeply and bend your knees until your thighs are parallel to the floor. Do *not* take a full bend; it could hurt your knees. To gauge how deep you are squatting, put a bench behind you and let your buttocks brush the bench lightly. Change directions without bouncing. Exhale while pushing with legs back up to starting position. Don't lock out; keep the legs slightly bent.

For the leg press, sit at a 45-degree leg press machine with your back flat against the pad and feet at a shoulder-width stance on a movement platform. Push out until legs are straight, then turn the safety pin to release the free movement. Inhale and slowly bend legs until thighs approach chest at the bottom position. Exhale while pushing back up to starting position, but don't lock knees out. Do not lower weight too fast.

STOMACH:	A: Seated leg kicks	3 giants sets, all to
	B: Standing leg raises	failure
	C: Sit-ups on slant board	

For the leg kicks, sit on edge of bench with legs hanging off the end and hands grasping the bench behind the buttocks to support the body. Begin with legs lifted and slightly bent. Without moving the upper body, pull legs into your chest by bending at hips and knees. Concentrate on lower abdominal muscles, holding flex position for a moment and then slowly extending to start position before repeating. Do in a fluid motion until failure. Blow out as your knees are coming in to chest—that's when you constrict the lower abs.

DAY TWO

BACK:	A: Lat machine, wide grip	2 sets front, 10 reps
		2 sets rear, 10 reps
	B: Lower cable rows to stomach	3 sets, 10 reps
	C: Bent-over rows, wide grip	4 sets, 10 reps

For lower cable rows, sit at a row station placing feet on pads and bending knees a bit. Grasp the close-grip handle with palms facing inward. Bend forward at the waist to stretch the lat and assume starting position. Pull the handle into the stomach area, simultaneously sitting upright without arching your back. Pause and stretch forward by bending your back once more before repeating. It's much like a rowing motion—you're sitting down, you're grabbing the handle, your knees are slightly bent on the pad. Your hands are going out and extending and bending from your hip area so your back is being pulled forward, then you're coming back and sitting up straight at attention. Bring the handles down to your belly button, then really flare and flex your back. Repeat.

SHOULDERS:	A: Seated military barbell press	3 sets, 10 reps
	B: Side dumbbell laterals	3 sets, 10 reps
	C: Barbell or dumbbell shoulder shrugs	3 sets, 10 reps
	D: Upright rows with barbell	3 sets, 10 reps

Shrugs are just what the name suggests—trying to get your shoulders up to your ears without bending your arms at all. With dumbbells, you stand up with the weights at the sides of your body. Squeeze your shoulders up and down. The more advanced can rotate during the motion. If you're using a barbell, hold it forward against your thighs. You can get a better range of motion with dumbbells.

For upright barbell rows, stand upright with knees slightly bent. Hold the bar with overhand grip just inside the shoulders. Begin with arms straight, then lift weight upward by bending elbows while keeping the bar close to the body until it touches under chin. Pause and lower.

BICEPS:	A: Bicep machine or preacher bench with barbell	2 sets close, 10 reps 2 sets wide, 10 reps
	B: Seated alternate dumbbell curls	3 sets, 10 reps
	C: Standing heavy curls with barbell	3 sets, 10 reps

With bicep machine, grab the bar (a close grip works the peak part of arm; a wide grip works inner part of bicep) and lean against the machine with armpits totally wedged against the pads and arms over the pads. Put *all* weight of chest against the pad so you can't cheat and use your back. Press elbows into pads, with arms fully extended down and grabbing onto the bar with underhand grip so fingers are facing you. Keep the elbows and back of trciceps against the pad at all times. Keeping arms straight, come up with the bar underneath the chin. Squeeze and constrict. Come back down just three-quarters of your range of movement; if you come down all the way you could hyperextend the muscle. Exhale coming up; blow out as you're going down. What you're doing here is absolutely isolating the bicep and working it fully. (Do the same exercise with a bar on a preacher bench at a a 45-degree decline. Don't swing your arms. Use a nice, fluid, slow motion. Constrict the muscle as you move up.)

| **CALVES:** | A: Standing calve raises
B: Seated calve raises | 3 supersets, 10 reps |

Use a standing calf raise machine after adjusting upper pads so weights are lifted when you stand upright on a floor platform. Place your hands on the upper handles and begin with knees straight and heels lowered to get a full stretch. Without bending the knees, exhale and flex the calf until you are standing tiptoe. Hold momentarily before inhaling as you lower back to stretch your calf in the starting position. Use moderately heavy weight. For best unrestricted movement, do this one in bare feet.

Advanced Weight Program

This individual has a foundation of at least two years' worth of weight training. Putting the proper rest interval into the program means that he or she will have to check the calendar to see which days are gym days. That's because it's a three-days-on, one-day-off, three-days-on, two-days-off regimen.

Note that at this plateau, he's down to two body parts per workout—each more thoroughly and intensively, allowing him to concentrate on his weak areas.

By now, he doesn't have to be reminded that he needs warmup (five minutes on bike) and cooldown (five minutes on stairs).

DAY ONE

CHEST:	4 supersets, 10 reps each	Incline bench press Incline dumbbell flyes
	4 supersets, 10 reps each	Flat bench press to neck Flat dumbbell flyes
	2 sets of 10 reps each	Decline dumbbell press, turn wrists in at top position

SHOULDERS:	Seated military press on machine or with barbell	3 sets, 10 reps
	Upright rows, barbell (narrow grip)	3 sets, 10 reps; vary position of grip after every set
	Alternate dumbbell front and side laterals Rear deltoid machine or bent-over rear side laterals	2 supersets of 10 reps each way
	Barbell or dumbbell shrugs	2 sets, 10 reps

CALVES:	Seated and standing calf raises	4 supersets: in, out, straight; use different foot positions

DAY TWO

BACK:	Wide-grip chin-ups	4 sets, 10 reps
	Wide-grip bent-over rows with barbell	4 sets of 10 reps
	Lat machine, wide grip	3 sets in front, 3 in back
	Lower cable rows	4 sets, 10 reps
	Dumbbell alternate rows	2 sets, 10 reps

TRICEPS:	Close-grip lat machine pushdowns Dumbbell overhead tricep extensions (elbows tucked into head).	4 supersets of 10 reps
	Seated tricep machine; Reverse close-grip pushdowns	3 supersets of 10 reps
	Alternate cable kickbacks	2 sets, 10 reps

DAY THREE

BICEPS:	Cable curls with bar Bicep machine or preacher bench	4 supersets: 2 close, 2 wide
	Seated alternate dumbbell curls	3 sets, 10 reps
	Concentrated curls	2 sets, 10 reps

LEGS:	Leg extensions, Smith machine ³/₄ squats	5 supersets, 10 reps each
	Leg press, leg curls	4 supersets, 10 reps each
	Sissy squats	2 sets to failure

STOMACH:	Sit-ups on slat board Ab crunch on bench Standing leg-raisers Sidebends on hyperextension	3 giant sets, all till failure

Nielsen's Junior Fitness Academy

After all that advanced stuff, I want to include this simple little program, which is very important to me. Fitness for kids is vitally important, no matter what activities we use to achieve it. Not all youngsters will take to the gym. But some will love it, and make it a lifetime program. Here's a basic workout for kids aged six and up.

Warmup is three to five minutes on bike. Cooldown is five minutes on stairs.

A: Leg extensions	2 sets of 10 reps
B: Tricep pushdowns	2 sets of 10 reps
C: Seated alternate dumbbell curls (for biceps)	2 sets of 10 reps
D: Shoulder side lateral	2 sets of 10 reps
E: Wide-grip lat machine pull-downs	2 sets of 10 reps

When I hand kids the printed workout, the notes at the bottom remind them that workouts will:

1. Build discipline
2. Help correct poor posture
3. Build strength
4. Build confidence and self-esteem
5. Help fight obesity
6. Help control high cholesterol
7. Exercise the most important muscle, the heart

21

Going All the Way

You're right. I'm an extremist.

As a pro bodybuilder, I've taken my own conditioning to the top one-tenth of one percent. As a nutrition counselor who walks what he talks, my daily menus look incredibly spartan compared with what everybody else on the block eats. As a human being, it actually *pains* me to see good people, successful people, smart people, educated people, kind people, thoughtful people being dragged down by not taking care of their bodies.

Why am I in so deep? Why do I push so far?

And what's the deal with that large number of people who go into the gym to lose a little flab, or to tone up a bit, or to regain some self-confidence—and wind up pushing farther than *they* ever imagined?

What's with all these extremists?

The answers are at the core of my message. Understanding what drives us extremists will help you comprehend the gifts of fitness—no matter what path you choose to achieve it, and whether or not you ever get within a mile of advanced weight training.

We're not talking muscleheads and gym rats—people for whom the gym is a pool hall, a place to hang out with their obsession. They do exist. Instead of being evenly yoked, they live only to pump iron.

We're talking accountants and broadcasters and business owners and housewives, people who live busy and fulfilling lives. Ninety-five percent of the time they never see a barbell. But for a half dozen hours spread through each week they are hard-core extremists, intensely devoted to a training regimen. They aren't just dabbling at the gym. They've moved upward from plateau to plateau to plateau without looking back. In most cases, no one is more surprised than themselves.

I rely on them to help explain what I'm about. I have to, because when I meet people outside the gym—in business, or socially, or in speechmaking—there's an almost invariable pattern. First, they want to see if I can walk and chew gum at the same time. Then they want to see if I can carry on intelligent conversation. Then, when I pass those tests, they come around a little bit. After all, *everybody* wants to be healthy. "You make a lot of sense, Peter," they'll say, "but why do you carry it *so far?* Who needs all those muscles?"

Let me get at it by telling you about the 25 percent. I can't exactly explain why, but about a quarter of my personal training clients wind up doing things that they never dreamed they'd do the day they walked in the door. I don't mean how many pounds of weight they lift, or whether some contest judges say they have the most symmetrical body on a stage. I mean in terms of a radically new attitude toward life.

Most come to me to lose a few pounds, or to firm up a bit, or because they're just tired of waking up tired. Almost everybody who lasts more than a few weeks benefits. They get into a program, they build a training foundation. All the physical things that happen—from metabolism to muscle tone—breed confidence and general well-being. For most people, that's plenty. But for this very large minority, this 25 percent, it's like they swallowed rocket fuel. Whoooooosh! Look out, world.

Part of it is this: The *real* competition in the gym is with yourself. That is the toughest, most rewarding, most meaningful competition in all of sport. You can set a world record every day. If you start out doing 10 reps with 50 pounds, then the day you do 10 reps with 55 pounds breaks the world record by 10 percent. If 10 minutes on the treadmill leaves you sucking wind, then the day you do 15 minutes you have *destroyed* the world record. It's the only reasonable way to look at it. Put two sprinters up against each other, or two racehorses, or two football teams. One of them might win without doing his best. It happens every day. The *only* way you can *ever* beat yourself is by doing your best.

And then this marvelous thing happens. Me against me becomes fun. Fun the way that rewarding, hard work is fun. Me against me becomes satisfying, the way real food is satisfying and candy isn't. And *your best keeps getting better.* On to the next plateau.

I couldn't list all the triggers that get pulled and send people into the gym for the first time. Some go because their spouse left them. Or because they figured out that they're losing money because their boss doesn't like fat people. Or because their nose is too big and their self-esteem is too small. Or because they've just realized that an idle body goes straight downhill with age. Or because they're fighting Crohn's disease and are absolutely infatuated with the idea of being alive inside a healthy body instead of being trapped in a crumbling prison. A million reasons, some of them serious and some of them trivial, make people take that first step through the door. Nobody, unless they're delirious, has those higher plateaus in mind on that first day.

When it starts happening, when your best keeps getting better, you finally look around one day and say: "What the hey; I think I *will* be the best that I can be." It spills out all over the place. In your personal life and your business life. You are the world champion in me vs. me. A lot of self-doubts go down that shower drain every day you work out. Who needs arrogance? Energy will suffice; and you have a surplus.

It's that energized, confident atmosphere that ignites the rocket fuel for the 25 percent. Stand back, because liftoff is going to be spectacular. And not very predictable.

Take my friend in Brooklyn. He was 60 pounds overweight. He regarded bodybuilding as a modeling show from Mars. It was the last thing he ever expected to get involved in; and when he came to me for PT, it was the last thing *I* ever expected him to be involved in. He built a foundation. He committed himself to a program. He shed the fat. He said, "Hey, this is fun, this is rewarding." And he took himself to the next plateau. Then—in the kind of blast-off behavior that no longer blows my mind—he decided to enter a bodybuilding competition. Not that he had changed his mind about bodybuilding contests. He just *wanted to prove something to himself.* And he got up on stage and won his class.

Or take the woman client who came to me many pounds over-weight. She was well-motivated and took to training like a bird takes to flight. She was disciplined and goal-oriented. But could I tell early on that she would be one of the 25 percent whose horizons and viewpoint would open up—BOOM—like the curtain on a play? No way. Until one day she revealed to me a new goal—not as a joke, not as a delusion, but as a calmly confident new goal. "I think I'd like," she said, "to pose for *Playboy.*" At this writing, she hasn't. But she *could.* The fact that training made her physically qualified to pose as a model or a *Playboy* subject isn't half as interesting as the fact that it made her want to do something so audacious. We're talking big-time change in ways a lot more important than a muscle here and there.

Do people make choices and chart paths differently when they're in top shape than when they're badly out of shape? Absolutely. Fitness and its relationship to mental attitude is potent, and complex. There is no question that fit people see things differently, and react differently. Making your best better physically can totally rearrange the way you interact in your daily life. I've seen it turn self-second-guessers into straightahead doers. When someone takes the extra step, becomes one of that 25 percent, the results sometimes approach rebirth.

So I'm an extremist. I came at weight training, like most people off the street, in terms of turning a negative into a positive. I've told you more in this book about the specifics that led me to the gym than I've ever told anyone. Really. Some of my best friends are going to be amazed.

But these are things you have to understand if this book is going to accomplish any of the things I want it to accomplish. There are plenty of books and magazines, some of them very bad and some of them very good, that run cover to cover with detailed exercise rou-tines. You can buy them at the corner drugstore. I had stacks of them down my grandmother's basement. But they're sterile. They don't tell the story. My own routines and programs are first-class. They're well-thought, based on 15 years of top experience, and they work. But no program is worth a penny unless you understand *why* you should be working out. Why you might become an extremist. Why you'll benefit even if you climb only half of the weight-training plateaus—or even if you just advance from couch potato to nutrition-conscious bicyclist.

I like to think the main reason I'm not a musclehead is I really believe that me vs. me is the competition that counts. I really do see world champions all over the place when I look around my gym. The body I live in is the result of the Peter Nielsen Me vs. Me Competition. Whether I ever win another trophy, or whether I ever did win a trophy, is not half as important as the fact that I am world champion of my own body. Nobody else can win that title. And I can't take away anybody else's.

I certainly can't win Chuck Robertson's title. Chuck is the *champion* extremist. He is in the top one percent of the 25 percent who decide to be the very best that they can be. My Crohn's problem looks like a head cold when you stack it up next to his spinal muscular atrophy (the Kennedy form, in medical terminology), a close cousin to Lou Gehrig's disease.

The traditional approach says a person with this disease shouldn't exercise. That tears down muscle—which is exactly what the disease is doing in its creeping, progressive march against the victim's body. But Chuck decided that instead of just putting his adversity in a closet and fading away, he would take charge and put it in front of him on a daily basis. He decided to learn all he could about nutrition and exercise. And he came to the gym to try to hold the disease in remission. We worked together, with his doctor's approval, on a fitness program.

In four to five months Chuck lost about 30 pounds of *fat*. He says he feels better than he has in many years. And when he lifts that arm and flexes, there it is: nothing that's going to win any hardware or wind up on the cover of a muscle mag, but an honest-to-God toned bicep. Nobody has to ask Chuck why *he* pushes so far.

In a few months I'll be meeting with one of the country's top specialists in diseases of muscular atrophy. We'll be going over the documentation of Chuck's physical therapy. Maybe we'll discover we've broken some new ground. If so, it'll fit a pattern of modern medical knowledge that is ironic: In a nation turned couch potatoes, health care professionals more and more are prescribing exercise for patients who used to be sent to bed for days or weeks. Everybody by now either has experienced, or has seen a family member experience, the new regimen of getting up and strolling the hospital corridor within hours after surgery. Exercise is a wondrous thing.

Another businessman, only in his 40s, came to me for physical therapy after two strokes. He was almost to the point of needing a wheelchair, and had lost much of his will to live. The doctors sent over his reports, let me know his limitations, and okayed a more aggressive approach. I designed a dumbbell and machine workout program for him and he went into the me vs. me competition. He went from a walker to a cane. Because of the passion in that internalized competition, and the strength it brought to his body, he is now living a much more normal life. He is stone intent on being the best he can be. And his best has gotten much better. Another extremist.

I don't *need* all those muscles, not the way Chuck needs the ones he's working on. But the only real difference between us is that I was blessed with body tissue that allows my best effort to produce musculature. I thank God every day for that, and for the opportunity to work with people like Chuck.

Yeah, I enjoy strutting my stuff in a bobybuilding competition. I *love* speaking to an audience that wants to know whether I can walk and chew gum at the same time. I thrive on the fencing matches that we call "business." Confidence, after all, is borderline cockiness. The fitter I am, the more it's there. That's true, I am convinced, of anybody.

What I enjoy most is getting that message through to other people. That's probably my ultimate reason for being an extremist: It helps get the message across.

Some of the people who hear it become extremists, too, and do audacious things. Fun and flippant things. Profound and moving things. Like deciding to pose for *Playboy*. Or making a stricken body take strides it isn't supposed to take.

22

Fighting a Flabby Future

Here's a conversation my friends and I never had 20 years ago, after a spirited session of street hockey in Brooklyn:

"Hey man! Are we gettin' our aerobics today, or what?"

"Yeah, man! Like, my heart's been at its ideal rate for an hour!"

"Yuh know, my basal metabolism rate is gonna be outa sight tonight."

We never had the conversation. It all would have been true, though. Street hockey was spontaneous, and we were having fun, but we were fitness freaks and didn't know it. We probably talked and yelled for a year without saying the word "fitness."

Nintendo hadn't been invented yet. Baseball was something kids played, not something that was on six TV channels seven nights a week. We weren't active because we were smart. We were active because *life* was active. Playing stickball and street hockey was like breathing.

In grade school, we went to phys ed classes *every day,* for 45 minutes. We had to. Today, in school district after school district, elementary physical education gets zero priority. In district after district, not even a weekly exercise session is required of all those high school kids who spend their lunch hours mainlining fat at the fast-food joints. Billions of dollars spent on education, and not five cents worth of intelligence about the human body trickles down to the students.

What in the world is going on here? We've got a major crime in progress and nobody's stopping it. It looks to me—as I think it would to anybody who analyzed the scene with an open mind—like we're breeding a generation of computer-literate cardiac cases. We spend 14 percent of our national wealth now on health care. That's with millions of Americans still alive who grew up active and spent their lives working with their hands. What do you suppose the bill is going to be when everybody who grew up with a joystick in one hand and a cheeseburger in the other hits middle age? Parents, and schools and every institution that has anything to do with our kids' well-being are going to have to answer some serious questions.

The days are long past when you could feed kids and let them run out the door to play, knowing the one thing they wouldn't be lacking when they came back was exercise. The more likely scenario now is slipping the kid a few bucks to buy his own grease and sugar, after which he or she plays computer games or watches music videos. And just when this huge fitness vacuum shows up among our youngsters, the schools practically walk away from the fitness business. Amazing.

I can't help thinking about my dog Angel, the gentle bull mastiff. There are laws, and proposed laws, around the country making it illegal for an owner to let a dog ride in the back of a pickup truck. People *argue* about these laws. The debate gets ink in the newspapers. Somebody gets *that* worked up about the health and safety of dogs, and I don't hear any outcry about the horror show that is our own kids' fitness! You tell me: If it's a $50 fine for letting your dog ride in the back of a truck, why isn't it a $5,000 fine for steering your 12-year-old child into a life of obesity, inactivity and future cardiac problems? Where are the priorities?

The boomers are getting a look at middle age now. That accounts for a big percentage of the mini-boom in exercise. You see a lot of affluent boomers at the health clubs, buying diet pills and workout videos, jogging. That's nice. But I haven't seen any statistics suggesting that the boomers are passing this newfound interest in fitness on to their kids. I know it's tougher these days to pass *any* kind of values on to youngsters. But we have to try harder. And we have to make fitness a whole lot bigger piece of the values picture for kids.

A young person probably will survive the wildest, trendiest music or hair style or language. He'll probably survive all the rites of passage. He'll probably get around the drug culture. Statistically, it looks like he'll probably dodge the AIDS epidemic. He'll probably endure the bad employment picture, though he might be living in your basement for a year or two. Somewhere down the line, he'll get past all the booby traps and be a normal, functioning, productive adult. But he has to do all that, and then live the next 60 years or so, *in the same body*. All of those scary things that your child must dodge or endure are real enough, but the fact is this: He's likely to have more sustained grief in his life because of his physical condition than because of all the rest of those obstacles put together.

Nobody has measured that, or written that, as far as I know. But think about it. There's a *long* road ahead after, say, age 21. More than two-thirds of the average American lifespan. Do you want your child running down that road on two cylinders half the time, and spending the other half the time in the repair shop? Of all the things you could pass on to your kids, shouldn't a passion for fitness be high on the list? Do you want your offspring *believing* that "life sucks, and then you die"? Nothing you hear on the street bugs me as much as that one. I can't prove it, but I *know* it's an attitude you almost never hear from somebody who takes fitness seriously. It makes sense if you have to drag your body out of bed and through the day. If you have energy to spare, and the positive force that comes with it, then it's a crock.

So how does a parent get the message across?

First, by not giving the opposite message. If a parent's own nutritional and exercise life is a disaster zone, then he or she is sending out the worst kind of signals loud and clear. Like everything else in parenting, suddenly you're not doing things just for yourself— you're doing them for those little people in the house who are all eyes and ears. You can't do anything about the million-dollar jock peddling junk food on TV, but you can do plenty about the mother and father peddling junk food in the living room. And you can keep your own role-model face from staring at the TV set for five hours a day.

Second, the good news is that the active state of mind is contagious among people living in close quarters. A lot of what passes for heredity is nothing but "inherited" *habits.* "Like father, like son" doesn't have much to do with genes. There are no "born tennis players"; but there are thousands of them who were born to tennis-playing families.

Third, more good news is that fitness can be a catalyst for a lot of other things you want to achieve as a parent. You hear a lot about "family values" these days. I'm not sure what that is. Your family's values might not be exactly the same as my family's values. But for sure, it all starts with the family being together. If you don't count TV watching—which I don't —family togetherness has become a rare event. Well, being active and being fit can make togetherness happen. A parent and a teen might have a tough time finding music they want to listen to together, but jogging, as one active example, is a different story. An entire family can hike together, or canoe together. Everybody in the canoe is getting fit; but they're also *talking,* sharing, understanding.

Grandparents need a footnote, by the way. Here's Grandpa, who spent 30 years unloading trucks and now spends two hours a day bending over and weeding his garden. For his age, he's probably more fit than 98 percent of the kids in America. He loves his grandchildren. So what does he do for the eight-year-old? He keeps him supplied with every video game known to man. The old smother-'em-with-love problem has its special twists in the '90s. Parents have to let the older generation know what's up. Put the video away, and let the kid go help Grandpa plant his zucchini.

Schools live in close quarters with kids for more hours a week than parents do. And somewhere along the line our schools have lost sight of producing a sound mind in a sound body. Educators are absolutely right when they throw a lot of blame for their failures back at parents. Parents who don't read generally have kids who don't read. Parents who are couch potatoes have kids who are couch potatoes. But the last time I looked, schools were still trying to teach kids to read. Meanwhile, many schools are doing no job, or at best a poor job, of teaching kids to be fit.

Start with doing no job at all. How can a school district not have a physical education requirement? It's insane. We're always looking to other countries for a rallying cry. If Germany or Japan teaches more math than we do, then it's a national disgrace for us. How about phys ed? All these countries that put more into their kids' brains put more exercise into their kids' bodies, too. Why aren't we upset about that? Why do we even need to look overseas? Study after study tells us what we already know: Our kids are inactive, and their bodies are paying the price. The real bill is going to come due in about 20 years. It seems obvious to me that we have to make phys ed a mandatory part of the curriculum in all of our schools.

That's just for starters. Then there's the matter of *what kind* of phys ed classes we offer. Here are three phys ed teachers I've run into. They're real people, but they're also types. You'll find them—and variations—in school gyms all around the country. Teacher A is a football coach, or an ex-football coach. He wants to teach 12- or 13-year-old kids that gang calisthenics are the way to stay fit. All together now, hup, two, three, four. Teacher B is a power lifter. He thinks the way to go is to teach kids to do short sets and add weight. For him, strength is where it's at. Teacher C is a woman gymnast. She opposes resistance training and is really into stretching. She obviously teaches quite a different way. It's as if we had some schools teaching that the Earth is flat, some that the Earth is round, and some that it's shaped like a kiwi.

We need to get everybody on the same page, the same frequency. You can't have kids from one school coming home and trying to bench press as much weight as they can, and kids from another school thinking that fitness means military push-ups. We need some shared standards and some shared goals. And then maybe —since it seems like everything in education sinks or swims on a national wave—phys ed departments would have the clout at budget time to get equipment and salaries that are needed for a good program.

When I talk to school assemblies—which I do about 50 times a year—I give a three-part message: nutrition, exercise and motivation. I tell them they may not be the *best* at throwing a baseball or running a mile, but by being active they can be *the best they can be*. I tell them that pigging out on junk food isn't half as pleasurable as feeling good and looking good because you eat right. Ninety-nine percent of the kids love it. Ninety-nine percent of the teachers love it. But nobody adds a phys ed requirement the next day. What happens the next day is that the PTA or the Band Boosters need to raise money. And how do they do it? By having all the moms send in layer cakes and peanut butter cookies to sell to the kids. Let's get serious!

Privately, many phys ed teachers tell me they just can't fight the bureaucracy. That there's no money for a program. That phys ed always has been and always will be the least glamorous and least respected job in the schoolhouse. That qualifications for leading a couple of hundred kids toward lifetime fitness are not always the qualifications that land the job.

These are big-time hurdles, and there are lots of dedicated teachers out there trying to jump them. They need some support from parents. That doesn't mean the Letter Club raising money so a few football players can wear NFL-type uniforms. It means a community's taxpayers saying: "We want our kids, all of them, to graduate with a sound mind in a sound body. We want our kids, after maybe $100,000 worth of education, to know nutritional poison as well as they know the multiplication tables. We want our kids to graduate with the cardiovascular health of an 18-year-old, not a 40-year-old. We want our kids to be thinking about fitness now, not after their first coronary."

That would be my dream—one big, squeaky wheel demanding and getting the grease it deserves.

Meanwhile, as a parent, do what you can on the homefront. Remember that togetherness and fitness go together like a bat and ball. If you really want to try something cool and far out and audacious, suggest to your teenage son or daughter that you launch a conditioning program together. Remember manual resistance—towels, broomsticks and Dynabands? *Great* conditioning for a teenager, as well as for you. And both of you need a training partner, so there you go.

If the idea of conditioning with mom or dad is just *too* far out for either child or parent, encourage your youngster to find another partner, to start a conditioning diary, and go at it. An amazing thing: I've seen parents encourage their kids to take piano lessons or art lessons, or to go to the museum or to build model airplanes, but I don't even need all the fingers on one hand to count the times I've seen a parent encourage a kid to work out! In fact, I've seen parents discourage it. "It'll stunt growth," they say. Or, "Growing bodies can't handle it."

That's pure nonsense. True, young people shouldn't be doing any weight resistance training above their head before the age of about 17. That leaves 99.9 percent of the conditioning arena open to teenagers. And there are a zillion ways to get children into an active, conditioning state of mind between the ages of six to 13, when they are most impressionable and likely to form lifelong habits. A few *pre-school* programs have designed activities around the idea of just getting together—including parents in the picture—and being active. Some specific resistance training can be appropriate as young as six or seven. Some sections of the country have junior fitness academies with formal workout programs.

You have no reason to fear harming a young child by encouraging him or her to try towel pulls, push-ups, sit-ups, running in place, riding a bike or playing soccer. Activity is the main thing, and aerobic activity will strengthen the youngster's heart, improve metabolism and encourage a good night's sleep. You want one of the really great workouts? Try a brisk session of jumping rope. And then remember that when you encourage your child to do it, there's a whole lot more going on than "going out to play."

Organized physical activity—whether it's a structured workout or playing on a soccer team—brings a dimension of mental development: discipline and a sense of responsibility. A child who is learning to take care of himself, to be more in tune with his or her body, is more likely to take care of and respect others. That comes from learning to respect himself, which is one of the great contributions of sports.

You can roll your eyes and say that sports is hideously overemphasized in this country, and you know something? I'd agree with you 100 percent. Except that "sports" is the wrong word in that sentence. *Watching* sports events and glamorizing the superstars is hideously overemphasized in this country. Some of the roundest couch potatoes in the universe think they're into sports. They're not. They're into watching. That's a different ballgame. Guzzling beer, holding a finger in the air, and screaming, "We're number one!" is not sports. Being into sports, for my money, means you play a team game, or you work out, or you run. The geeks who guzzle beer and watch 50 games a week seldom do any of those things. And they give sports a bad name.

Maybe that's why soccer intrigues me as a fitness sport for kids, even though I never played the game. Hundreds of thousands of youngsters across the country play this sport—even though not one parent in 100 ever played it, and even though you need a satellite dish and a foreign language translator to pick it up on your TV. It requires minimal equipment, gets a maximum number of kids involved, and involves vigorous exercise. Kids love it. That should tell you something.

It may sound farfetched, but the discipline I learned at a young age—lifting weights under Julie's guidance—has carried through my adult life. Even the street hockey is a part of that picture. We played hard; we had rules. The karate lessons helped make me more open, more communicative, more self-confident—even though I hated going to class every week. Actually, there's a sport or exercise out there waiting for every youngster, one he or she will look forward to. You just have to find the right match. It might be something foreign to you (just look at all those soccer players), so if your boy doesn't want to be a fullback just like Dad, don't push him into it.

It is so important that we find ways of increasing the active state of mind among our young people. I regard that as the most important thing I do. In my new home state of Michigan, I'm active on the Governor's Fitness Council. I talk to school superintendents and athletic directors. I'm working to get a coordinated fitness policy in all the schools in my home county.

We need a few hundred thousand other people pushing in the same direction.

Part Four:

The Eye of the Tiger

23

Learning to Learn

It all comes down to this: If you don't have that mental toughness, that Eye of the Tiger, then your total fitness package will come unwrapped. Knowledge alone isn't enough. There are overweight nutritionists and out-of-shape physiologists. There are doctors who smoke cigarettes. They all know better. They all lack the Eye of the Tiger.

If you read and absorb every word in this book—in a hundred books—about nutrition and exercise, all you will have gained is information. Having the Eye of the Tiger isn't just about collecting data. For that matter, it isn't just about nutrition and exercise. It's about focusing so intently on what's real, on putting one foot in front of the other in a *positive* direction, that your steps will take you where you want to be. That applies to all three of the big ones: health and fitness, relationships, career. Most people don't focus. Their steps are aimless. And instead of living quality lives, they just exist.

I said you must train your mind before you can sustain a nutrition and exercise regimen. What I want to say in this chapter is the closest I can come to telling you how to do that. I can't hand you the Eye of the Tiger the way I can hand you things I know about protein and carbos and supersets. You have to reach out and get that mental toughness yourself. But it's within everybody's grasp.

That's because mistakes and adversities are the raw material. If you can't find any mistakes and adversities in this world, you *really* are out of focus. Most of us find them every day. Our mistakes, other people's mistakes. Our adversities, other people's adversities. Little ones, medium-sized ones, monsters. There's enough raw material out there to make us all so mentally tough that we could cut steel just by thinking about it. What you need to do is take all the mistakes and adversities, grind them up, and recycle them into opportunities for positive action.

Yes, we are talking about positive thinking. Big-time positive thinking. I've built a transformer someplace in my gut that takes every negative ion in my body and gives it a positive charge. If you're cynical about that kind of talk, hang around a minute. Because I think the cynics are the real Pollyannas. People who have the Eye of the Tiger confront their mistakes and adversities head-on. People with the negative, life-sucks-and-then-you-die attitude spend their days whining and dodging the troubles they see lurking all around them. *They* are the ones who need a reality check.

Think about this: Most anyone would agree there are three big places you can have setbacks—in your health, in your personal relationships, in your finances. I had a debilitating disease that almost killed me. I had a personal relationship that left scar tissue on my heart. And then I lost nearly $200,000, virtually all my money, when my first real business deal went sour. All this by my mid-20s. What do I have now, at 31? More energy per day than there are hours on the clock. Several businesses and several careers. A marriage with a wonderful woman who has a thousand golden attributes—including the Eye of the Tiger. Is this all an accident? No way. You could give me Yale University for Christmas and I wouldn't learn as much as I did from those three setbacks.

The mind-boggling flip side of that picture is that the world is crammed full of people who don't learn from their mistakes and their adversities. Every day a few million learning opportunities get swept into the closet, like dusty old textbooks. Instead of confronting them head-on with a positive-thinking mental toughness, the negative thinkers sidestep every single learning opportunity. And they land knee-deep in crud.

What do I see as an example? I see a Crohn's patient a few months out of the hospital—after almost exactly the same miserable, devastating experience I went through—trying to eat pizza. Hamburgers. Hot fudge sundaes. Martinis. He comes to me for nutritional counseling, and what he really wants is a strategy for getting this stuff into his stomach. What's *wrong* with this picture? Maybe the doctors should bottle a foot or two of intestine in formaldehyde for every surgical patient and make them carry it around, just to remind them of reality.

A Crohn's patient who wants to pretend that he can knock down a martini-and-burger lunch is doing exactly what most people do with adversity in every corner of their lives, big and small. It's easier—in the short term—to shunt the problem aside, to deny it, to avoid it. And if you're a negative-thinking person that's only logical, *because you have nothing to bring to the problem.* What's needed is to set an adversity right on the examining table, at eye level, the way Chuck Robertson did, and say: "OK, let's see what we have here, and figure out what we can do with it." *That* is learning from an adversity or a mistake. *That* is the Eye of the Tiger. *That* is so much mental toughness that I wish I could bottle it and give it to the world.

It has to do with getting past the sorrow, the self-pity, the resentment, the temper tantrums, the why-me syndrome? In my case I had to learn that a family will continue with their lives whether you are sulking in a corner or not. That your girlfriend will finally get disgusted with your negative, pessimistic personality. That the other guys on the block will get tired of hearing about your bad deck of cards and go play hockey without you. Long before Julie Levine had me looking in mirrors to check out progress on my muscles, I had to look in a mirror to check out progress on my life. Once I did that and realized that the guy staring back at me did *not* have it worse than anyone else in the universe, and that he was the *only* person who could solve my problems, then I was lit. I had the spark. I was ready to try to take control of my life.

My own adversities were a blessing in disguise, because they were big-time. The difference between having small adversities and big adversities is the difference between being in a class of 100 students and having your own personal tutor. I'll never know if I would have been smart enough to collect my advanced degree if I hadn't been told, at 15, that I might die. I'd probably be in line this afternoon at the pork shop. That's why I can say in total honesty that if I could do it all over, I wouldn't have it any other way. My life would have gone in an entirely different direction. Besides eating sausages every morning, I'd be more complacent, more naive. I'd be more cocky and self-centered. I'd have my priorities and values all screwed up. I know I wouldn't be married, wouldn't be thinking with as much business savvy as I do.

In recent years I've figured out that thousands of the most successful people have been blessed with serious adversity. I've met dozens of people whose health and wealth hit the top of the scale—but who also have humility, personality and a commitment to a positive lifestyle. What do they have in common? Ninety percent of them have been through some kind of trauma. They've seen both sides of the river. They learned, and they remembered. They have the Eye of the Tiger.

It starts with a spark, an electrifying flash of reality. Sparks come from a million sources. You don't have to experience trauma; you don't have to be struck by lightning. Seeing someone on the street with a smile on his face and only one leg on his body could light a spark. I know I light sparks with many low-esteem kids when I speak at schools and explain that this muscle guy was, at their age, one very imperfect specimen. Ninety percent of the people who come to my gym for the first time are driven there by scary sparks—or by wake-up calls masquerading as sparks. A divorce, or a threat of divorce. A sudden realization of mortality. I've had first-timers come *directly from the doctor's office,* carrying their off-the-graph cholesterol readings.

But it takes more than a spark. It takes a strong flame, because people and events will be trying to blow out the fire every day. That is the trick to motivation, to what I am trying to pass on to you. Sparks can come easy. Flames are a tougher piece of business. Most sparks are *so* fragile. People *want* to take control of their lives. They accumulate the knowledge, and they keep trying to fan the spark into a flame, but the fire never takes hold. You can't believe how many people come to me for nutrition counseling and, after I tell them the score, they say: "I *know* that." Fifty percent of their calories are coming from fat. I'm telling them that they're killing themselves. And they're saying: "I *know* that."

All I can conclude is that they don't really *know* anything. They've got some data stored in their head, all right, but they haven't really learned a thing. Not from their mistakes. Not from other people's mistakes. All this raw material going to waste. There's a level of knowledge that doesn't have anything to do with facts and numbers, and they don't have it. Live and learn? Not really. Not for most people, not most of the time.

You see, having adversity in your life isn't the secret. We all have at least some of that. Sometimes even mega-adversity or world-class mistakes aren't enough. Many people get trapped in a fail-fail-fail syndrome when the handwriting is right on the bridge of their nose. The guy with 20 straight failed relationships, for example, who says he's "still looking for the right girl." It doesn't occur to him that he should be looking in the mirror for the right *guy*, that maybe it's time for some positive change.

The secret, obviously, is the capacity to learn real-world lessons. To establish radio contact between abstract facts you "know" (fat is a bad thing) and personal facts you are avoiding (you can't see your shoes). To look in a realistic mirror instead of a circus mirror that reflects only what you want to see. It's like that second lens I asked you to use when you look at the food you eat. A triple chocolate parfait sundae with whipped cream and coconut is a circus sideshow. Mega-doses of fat and cholesterol are the reality. Like the man said, "I already *know* that." But does he, really, if he's eating it? And what in the world does he see when he looks in the mirror?

We like to think that little kids live in a fantasy world and us big people are out there plowing our way through the real world. I'm not so sure. Little kids don't have to be hit by a truck to figure out that playing in the street is a bad idea. Why should you have to be diagnosed with cancer before you'll give up cigarettes? Why should you need a heart attack to truly understand what obesity and poor cardiovascular fitness can do to you? Some people need the big wake-up call. Some people have the capacity to learn.

Let me give you *my* definition of a smart person: someone who learns from *other* people's mistakes and adversities. Throw away the college entrance exams—this is a person with a mind that works in the real world. It's as simple as that. On the streets of life, he or she will play on the sidewalk instead of in the passing lane. Smart person. Am I a smart guy? I guess so, because I now learn from other people's mistakes and adversities every day. I wasn't always that smart.

Your own mistakes can be learning experiences only if they're not too big. The bigger the mistake, the more a person is likely to learn—but the more likely that it's too late.

When my Dad got sick, he talked about taking a little more time off from work, partying less, retiring early. He decided to quit smoking, finally, and made it a point to tell me. Then he got an oxygen tank, just before the doctor called to say that Pete Nielsen had maybe a month to live. I can't tell you how hard it was to tell my Dad that his mistake was too costly. He had gotten the scare, made the commitment. But he was a day late and a dollar short. He died in *less* than a month, at 49.

Another statistic, another lesson.

If you want the Eye of the Tiger, you have to start making the connections. Personally. Not in a textbook. Not in concept. *In your own life*. That's what real learning is about. We're talking permanent change here. There is no quick fix. There are no substitutions on this menu. No excuses. Garbage in, garbage out. That's reality, and you've got to *get real*. If you want to light a flame that will stay lit, then you've got to deal honestly with the only statistic you can do anything about. You. Your body, your blood pressure, your musculature, your priorities, your values. Society puts a fantasy menu in front of you every day. It's all junk food and remote controls. When you have mental toughness, you'll reject all of it.

"Mental toughness" sounds so macho, but it's not. Macho is fantasy—flawless and indestructible is not reality. Macho means insecurity and some kind of inferiority complex. Mental toughness means learning from mistakes, being honest with yourself. You've got to sweat, but you've also got to cry. You've got to be truthful, and see what's really in the mirror instead of what you'd like to see. You've got to accept that that this is the deck you've been dealt, and that changes are in order. When you are mentally tough, you have nothing to prove. You know what you have to do, you have a game plan, and you're going to do it. That's the Eye of the Tiger.

Positive thinking is the cutting edge of mental toughness. It will make you the best that you can be. And—if you are a lost, negative soul—you'll be amazed what a positive attitude can do for your relationships with other people. It only takes a minute to spread bad news. If what you project in a room—socially or at work—is pessimism, if your thinking and your conversation is dominated by what *can't* be done instead of what *can* be done, then it'll only take a minute for everybody to wish you were somewhere else.

We all like to hear good things about ourselves, and I hear two things that make me feel good. When people meet me, they say they're surprised that I'm deeper than the cosmetic look that I project (as if muscles and intelligent life couldn't co-exist). And they say that my positive outlook is *addictive* (as if anyone could get high on a negative outlook). *I'm* addicted to positive vibes in other people. Sometimes you don't even have to talk to someone to know. You can practically see the electricity. It's the opposite of the negative person. With them, you can practically hear the whine.

Do I ever get mad? Of course. Often. Do I get frustrated? Of course. Do I have negative thoughts? Thousands. I work a lot of them out in the gym. Don't forget that one of the very biggest benefits of *physical* fitness is *mental*. You may never touch a barbell in your life, but there are other ways. All those runners you see along the road are burning more than calories. Any good exercise will do. Fitness is so good for the mind that I think I see a correlation between flabbiness and negative, angry behavior. I can't prove it, but I believe it. It *is* a package.

Negative and positive go together like love and hate. Energy is energy. You can use it positively or you can use it negatively. It's the difference between nuclear power and a hydrogen bomb. When you've got your package together, you'll always be looking to harness and channel the energy of a situation in a positive direction.

Cindy and I were at a gathering where someone dear to me collapsed with a heart attack. She turned blue. Her eyes rolled back in her head. She stopped breathing. There were 16 other guests, so there were 18 of us who were frightened and charged with energy.

Sixteen people started wringing their hands and running in circles like ants on hot coals. Cindy and I helped the victim to the floor. Cindy ran and called 911 while I started giving the victim resuscitation. Everybody had the same energy. Two of us were channeling it in a positive direction.

That's a simple, graphic example of what I mean by meeting a situation head-on, evaluating it, and deciding whether to march through it, over it, under it, or around it, choosing the most positive course. It doesn't have to be anything as dramatic as a heart attack. But no matter the type of obstacle—and needing to turn your physical and nutritional life around *is* an obstacle —you need to meet it head-on, one-on-one. How you respond is a me vs. me challenge, just like in the gym. You are the sculptor, you are in control—if you take a positive approach.

In any situation where you're scared, on the other side of scared is success. Success vs. failure is a 50–50 proposition. They're separated by such a thin line, and often that line is fear. Too many people fail even to light the flame because they're afraid they'll fall short of perfection. That's silly. The Eye of the Tiger isn't about being the best in the world, or even about being the best on the block. It's about being the best you can be. No more, no less. Once the flame is lit, it's often a surprise just how good that turns out to be.

Let's say you've got the spark, and you're trying to light the flame and keep it going for the rest of your life. Let's say you've had some long conversations with yourself about making an effort to channel all your energies in a positive direction. Let's say you've done your homework, and you know a complex carbohydrate from a T-bone steak. Let's say you believe you're ready to make a commitment. Let's say you want to develop the Eye of the Tiger, but you need some training wheels. Where do you get the determination to get the thing rolling?

Focus. Focus. Focus. On what? On reality. Determination comes when a person first becomes realistic, and then sets realistic goals. Don't kid yourself. You've got to prioritize. If you are a couch potato, you're goal isn't to win Mr. Universe next fall. Your goal might be to be able to walk comfortably to the park and back next month.

Write down your short-term and long-term goals. Make the

timespan realistic. Don't be like the prospective clients who come to me after 30 years of abusing their bodies and expect me to make them into Venus or Adonis in 60 days. *Get real.* You've got the rest of your life to be your best. Start out by being better tomorrow than you are today—not by trying to be where you ought to be in six months or a year.

Get on a low-fat diet. Get the cardiovascular system going with a modest exercise regimen, like walking. Then escalate. Be better every week, every month, every year. Build your mental toughness and physical condition side by side. Accept the fact that your health is the most valuable thing you ever will have, or lose. Recognize that you are confronting the thing that people fear most: *change.* Permanent, life-altering change.

Put it all out on the table—your hopes, your fears, the reality of your fitness, where you want to be. Analyze the situation and say: "What do we have here? And what's the best way to approach it." Don't look behind you to see who else is in the picture, because nobody can do this but you.

When you get that far, you'll start to see and hear things.

You'll get a glimpse of a determined, realistic you. That's the Eye of the Tiger struggling to be born.

And you'll hear a voice in your head, asking: "How *bad* do you want it?"

Get used to the voice. It'll never go away.

Acknowledgments

This is a book, not the Academy Awards. That's good, because I need a couple of minutes to mention quite a few people who played a role in the good things that have happened to me. Life's like that, if you get up off the couch and dive into each day with energy and a positive attitude. Next thing you know, you've gathered a cast of thousands.

I'm a religious person, something you may or may not have picked up while reading this book. My beliefs run deep. I certainly didn't try to hide them. I also didn't want to confuse any issues here, or lose any readers whose religion—or lack of it—isn't the same as mine. Maybe some day I'll get a chance to do a book that explains how a muscle specialist with a lingering Brooklyn accent finds incredible strength every day in his relationship with God. For now, let me just start out by acknowledging Him.

I'd also like to acknowledge the hard work and sweat equity that the Crohn's and Colitis Foundation of America has devoted to finding a cure, and to providing support.

And, in no particular order, I need to mention a few first-class people. Some of them you met in these pages, and some you didn't:

Julie Levine, who showed me that it was more than a hobby.

Yvonne Wind, for wisdom beyond her years.

Robert Figliulo, my best friend and the finest mechanic on Long Island; and Walter Gatto, who was there beginning in kindergarten.

Dan Lurie, who got me to Belize.

Paul Jarbara, a key link in my chain—thanks for the intro that led me to Detroit.

Tom Celani, who—by letting me make a few bucks endorsing fruit juice—kept me alive in the early days in Detroit, and who has never stopped believing in me.

Rod Welsh, first a friend and second somebody who made my vitamins a Blue Light Special.

Charlie Baughman, who stepped forward when things looked really grim.

Calvin Mackey, my accountant, whose numbers let me open some doors—even when I hadn't paid him yet for the numbers.

Peter Kupelian, Mark Cantor and Mark Fishman, attorneys who took care of all kinds of details that I couldn't have found with a microscope.

Chuck Robertson, for his friendship, inspiration and constant reminder that Me vs. Me is the greatest competition of all.

Cheh Low and Steven Downs of the WNBF, and Andy Bostinto of its amateur division, the NGA, for all they've done to make sure bodybuilding is about muscles and not about drugs.

Eli Zaret, Fred McLeod, Bruce Kirk and Kathy Adams—on-the-air talents who did so much off the air to make me feel at home in front of a camera.

Peter Ginopolis, a great restaurateur and host—but who knows how to grill a serious whitefish without butter.

Russ Pauling, the first to license my name on a gym.

Bill Haney and Terry Livermore of DMB&B in Bloomfield Hills, who showed me how the pros put a package together.

Darryl and Erma Wood, the best Bible teachers in the upper Midwest.

Pastor Mitchell Maloney, who constantly reminds me of the importance of being evenly yoked.

James Bragman, D.O., diplomat, American Board of Internal Medicine, for reading parts of the manuscript.

BestAmor Edna Nielsen and Nana Antoinette Romanzi—the Danish and the Italian grandmothers, my links with tradition.

John DuFermont, my right arm and alter ego at the sports medicine clinic.

Buzz Silverman, a genuine confidant and an incredibly savvy businessman.

Spencer Partrich, valued mentor and living proof that you can become a terror in the gym after five decades of avoiding it.

Tom Ferguson, the writer who saw to it that it's the real me who's talking in these pages.

Sandy and Leon Karash, true friends and supporters—just the opposite of every old New York comedian's idea of in-laws.

Kim, a talented sister whose dreams could be seen in her eyes the first time she sang with the band, and who yelled the loudest when I went on stage.

Pete Nielsen, who was with us long enough to make me a man, and who paid the biggest price to show me the way.

Marie Nielsen, whose pasta and love could have nurtured a dozen more of us kids.

There are many others, of course, valued links in the human chain that defines our time on Earth. They are there for all of us, if we keep our bodies fit enough to find them, and our minds positive enough to give something in return.